Dr Libby's

Beauty From The Inside Out

Enhance The Gifts Nature So Graciously Gave You

Dr Libby Weaver

Disclaimer

The contents of this book are for information only, and are intended to assist readers in identifying symptoms and conditions they may be experiencing. This book is not intended to be a substitute for obtaining proper medical advice and must not be relied upon in this way. Always consult a qualified doctor or health practitioner. The author and publisher do not accept responsibility for illness arising out of the failure to seek medical advice from a doctor. In the event that you use any of the information in this book for yourself or your family or friends, the author and the publisher assume no responsibility for your actions.

Published by Little Green Frog Publishing Ltd
www.littlegreenfrogpublishing.com

ISBN: 978-0-473-25304-2

Registered Reader

Congratulations on purchasing *Beauty from the Inside Out*. The science and our understanding of the impact that nutrition and lifestyle choices have on our bodies are constantly changing, as colleagues in the research world continue to make breakthroughs.

By purchasing this book, you qualify for our Registered Reader program. Our aim with this Registered Reader program is to ensure that we are able to keep you abreast of the latest developments in health and well-being, as well as provide you with a touch point to continue to motivate you to achieve the goals you desire for your health and body.

Please become a registered reader by visiting:

www.drlibby.com/bioresources

Also by Dr Libby Weaver

Accidentally Overweight

Rushing Woman's Syndrome

Dr Libby's Real Food Chef, with chef Cynthia

For Christopher with huge gratitude for the beautiful love and life we share

and

For my dear Mum and Dad with huge gratitude for being such beautiful parents and treasured friends

Table of Contents

My mission is to educate and inspire, enhancing people's health and happiness, igniting a ripple effect that transforms the world.

SHINE

intransitive verb

1: to emit rays of light
2: to be bright by reflection of light
3a: to be eminent, conspicuous, or distinguished <*shines* in mathematics>
b: to perform extremely well <when will stocks really *shine* again?>
4: to have a bright glowing appearance <his face *shone* with enthusiasm>
5: to be conspicuously evident or clear

transitive verb
1a: to cause to emit light
b: to throw or direct the light of
2: to make bright by polishing

Origin of SHINE
Middle English, from Old English *scīnan;* akin to Old High German *skīnan* to shine and perhaps to Greek *skia* shadow
First known use: before 12th century

Related to SHINE
Synonyms: beam, radiate, ray
Related words
blaze, burn, fire, flame, gleam, glimmer, glint, glisten, glister, glitter, glow, luminesce, sheen, shimmer; blink, coruscate, flare, flash, flicker, luster (*or* lustre), scintillate, spangle, sparkle, twinkle, wink, winkle; beat (down), glare; brighten, illuminate, illumine, irradiate, light, lighten; bedazzle, blind, daze, dazzle

noun
1:brightness caused by the emission of light
2: brightness caused by the reflection of light: luster <the *shine* of polished silver>
3: brilliance, splendor <has a *shine* about her>
4: fair weather: sunshine <rain or *shine*>
5: track, caper —usually used in plural
6: liking, fancy <took a *shine* to him>
7: a polish or gloss given

Merriam-Webster's Collegiate Dictionary

Let your light shine

What dulls your shine?

As research for this book, I asked some precious humans what they felt "dulled their shine". Here is what they said:

Alcohol
Processed food
Stress
Sugar
Bad sleep
Worry
Gluten
Dairy
MSG
Self-criticism
Pressure
Energy drinks
Family issues
Hunger
Urinary problems
Reproductive problems

Antibiotics
Boredom
Rejection
Greasy food
Gossip
Bullying
Toxic cosmetics
Can't warm up, cold in the bones
Too much to do
Rushing food
People pleasing
Over-eating
Comfort eating
Unexplained weight gain
Aerosols
Bad skin
Colds and illnesses
Comparing self to others
Disrupted menstrual cycle
Too much technology
No solitude
No sunshine
    Bad lighting, and/or dark/damp living conditions
False accusations
Violent and angry behaviour
Criticism
Overwhelm
Peer pressure eating/drinking
Drugs
Guilty eating

Cleaning products
The news
Disappointment
Dehydration
Air conditioning
Shock
Fear
Anxiety
Hurt
Surgery
Vitamin deficiency
Contraceptive pill
Heavy periods
Painful periods
Jealousy
Skipping meals

Just to name a few ...

Do you relate to any of these? If so, which ones? It might be lovely and also helpful for you while you read this book to keep a journal. You may have a notebook on hand that you can use, or buy yourself a new one with a colour or image on the cover that you like. Capture what arises for you while reading this list. What do you feel dulls your shine? Knowing from the start where you want to focus as this book unfolds can help guide you to make some new choices that help support your well-being and your shine!

For beautiful eyes, look for the good in others; for beautiful lips, speak only words of kindness; and for poise, walk with the knowledge that you are never alone.

Audrey Hepburn

INTRODUCTION

Beauty really is an inside job. How many of us stop to consider that our outer layer is merely a reflection of inner processes, completely reliant on the health of the 50 trillion cells that you are made of? And the health of those cells is impacted by everything from the food you eat, the nutrients present or missing from your blood, and the hormones and messages your body makes based on whether your thoughts are fearful or loving. Think about that.

When most people think about improving their appearance, they usually focus on a product, another "quick fix". Yet when you consider that the skin cells on your face are a small percentage of the total number of cells in the whole body, it seems crazy that we don't spend more time getting the majority of the cells functioning optimally, leading us to the outcomes we seek.

Throughout these pages, we will decipher beauty like never before, and you will be guided on which levers to pull to help you create, recognize, and deeply appreciate your beautiful shine. The chapters vary in length from one another, not based on importance but simply because some topics require more explanation. We will explore your outer world — the food you choose, the nutrients you ingest, hydration, posture, movement, skin, hair and nails — and we will delve into your inner world of sex hormones, stress hormones, detox, digestion, elimination pathways, thyroid and pituitary functions, and how both worlds relate to your sparkle. This is not a book teaching you how to cleanse, tone and moisturise. We will look into the superstar beauty support that sleep offers, and at ways to make sure your sleep is restorative. I will explain what your body needs to create lovely nails, lustrous hair, sparkling eyes, and clear, luminous skin, and you will also be guided to deal with very specific bumps in the road, such as dark circles under the eyes, eczema, pimples, and hair that is falling out, just to name a few. Just as importantly, we will explore your inner world, by taking a heart-opening look at your emotional landscape because, for many, that is where the real elixir is.

So, this book takes you on a journey through the physical aspects of your health and beauty, but also the emotional, guiding you to experience and deeply appreciate your own radiant beauty from the inside out!

Inner health and transformation has the power to affect your outer beauty by improving the health of your skin, transforming the shape and movement of your body, and allowing you to express a radiance that inspires those around you.

You will notice throughout the book that when I talk about beauty, I will often refer to it as your "shine" or your "sparkle", as for me beauty is a light in the heart. It is radiance. It is luminous and joyful, and it is inside every single precious human. Yet, regardless of her appearance, ask any women if she thinks she is beautiful, and almost all women reply no, or ask you if you think she looks OK. Many women get teary if you compliment them. Let this book help you unlock and deeply appreciate your shine and allow you to share your gifts with the world, for if you knew who you really are, you would be in awe of yourself. As Oscar Wilde wrote "One does not see anything until one sees its beauty" — a statement that is oh-so-true when it comes to human beings being able to see themselves through the eyes of a beloved, rather than years or decades of comparing themselves to others. Remember, if you struggle with insecurity, it may be because you are comparing your behind-the-scenes with every-one else's highlight reel, a sentiment that has been so beautifully shared by Steve Furtick.

There is so much beauty on offer to us 24/7, inside us, around us, and shining from us. For so many, a veil just needs to be lifted so you can experience your own radiance. Let's see what we can do!

As a society, our relationship with beauty is in crisis. We are told that beauty exists only in certain forms, images, and at certain ages. We can feel bombarded with images that lead us away from our own unique beauty and encourage us to try to look like someone else rather than become and accept more of who we are. While adults can be affected by such messages, these messages can be particularly damaging to children and teenagers who so desperately want to be loved, approved of, considered special, and seen as beautiful. From an emotional maturity perspective, wanting to fit in is natural at this age, and many teens today will tell you they believe they have to look good to fit in.

Equally damaging can be the perception that beauty is unattainable beyond a certain age. In this era, youth is worshipped, and many attempt to deny the aging process. Yet due to the advances of medicine, hygiene, and technology, we are living longer and longer (I will say more about *quality* of life later), and the possibility of people alive now living to be 120 or 150 years of age is not far-fetched. Yet, by current definitions of youthful beauty, this means that for less than about 15 per cent of your life, you'd tick the box for having half a chance to be beautiful. You must be joking!

With more time on this magnificent planet can come wisdom, emotional maturity, spiritual growth, and a trust and knowing from past experience that no matter what happens, it is all part of a bigger picture that sometimes you can't see when the tough stuff is going on. Why wait until you are older to learn this and then live from this trusting space? Regardless of age, however, if you are full of conflicts and tension, and are resistant to emotional growth, you tend to feel flat, doubt yourself, and have tougher challenges in relationships. Each stage of life offers us beautiful opportunities to experience our own inner and outer beauty.

THE MYSTERIOUS PULL OF BEAUTY

Whether it's acknowledged or not, most women want to be beautiful. Everyone wants to look good. Yet most people believe they need to change something or even a multitude of things before beauty is possible — and even then it's only a maybe!

So why does beauty seem to have this mysterious pull? Why are we attracted to what we consider to be beautiful? Why is it that you seem to become a powerful magnet for people and opportunities when you, yourself, feel beautiful? The reason beauty calls to us is because it arises from love, which is itself the most nourishing and desired force in life. Beauty is the consequence of love. Think about that. And beauty therefore announces the presence of love, to which we are inherently drawn.

Would you believe me if I told you that your experience of your own beauty is dependent on you loving yourself? I am not saying that you just need to affirm that you love yourself and it's a done deal. Every human's greatest fear is that they are not enough, and that if they are not enough they won't be loved. We are born this way. It is Human Psychology 101, and it is hardwired into a part of our nervous system that we cannot access with our thoughts. The reason not being loved is our greatest fear, and one with which we are born, is because without love a human baby dies, as someone has to care for us enough to feed us and provide us with clothing and shelter. Other animals can forage for food and find shelter and survive. So this is not some artificial construct that develops over time — it is hardwired into our nervous system at our most fundamental level.

However, as adults, while a life with love in it is delicious, it is not critical on a physical level to our survival, as we have the ability to obtain our own food, clothing, and shelter. Yet most adults still believe unknowingly that they must be loved, or liked, or fit in — whatever language you feel most comfortable using — to survive, which drives their desires and behaviour; hence their pursuit of beauty.

But, if you are not careful, you may spend your whole life searching externally for love when it is, in fact, internally on offer to you. Any time you choose to remember, what you were born knowing: that you are beautiful and so very precious. You simply unlearned and stopped believing this. Let me remind you of what your heart already knows.

It is very difficult to be patient and kind with yourself and others, when you are filling yourself with stimulants such as too much caffeine and refined sugars, and eating a diet high in processed foods that is virtually devoid of nutrients.

Dr Libby

Chapter 1

Beautiful Foods:

the powerful impact of real food
on your beauty

When it comes to your physical health and beauty, the foundation stone is the way you nourish yourself through the foods you choose. Nothing, and I mean nothing, compares to what real food offers your physical health and radiant self. When it comes to food, Nature gets it right, while human intervention can get it very wrong. Let me explain why this matters so much and why it is essential that you take good care of the way you nourish yourself.

Nutrition is one of the most debated topics in the health arena. People are constantly looking at new ways they can improve their nutrition, and consequently their health and how they look, but unfortunately there are huge amounts of misinformation out there. Theories about the healthiest way to eat abound, yet what science has firmly established is the protective benefits of a largely plant-based diet.[1] Whole foods contain all of the foods' vitamins and minerals, as well as their natural plant compounds which are known to support human health. After all, it is nutrients that keep us alive. Really think about that. Without nutrients, we die, and we get our nutrients primarily through the foods we choose. Eating real food is about all of the perks you get (for example, nutrient density), but it is also about what you miss out on — the potentially harmful substances in processed food that can disrupt your body's natural rhythms, biochemistry, communication systems, and hormonal systems. When you eat mostly real food, you omit most of the artificial colours, flavours, sweeteners, preservatives, and additives that can be present in processed foods. You also miss out on ingredients that have been bleached and/or pummelled so that any nutrients that may have been in the original food have to be added back synthetically for that food to even have any goodness. Imagine that! And yet most people eat these foods daily without giving any thought to what they might be doing to their insides ... and hence their outside appearance. You cannot fill up on stimulants, such as too much caffeine and refined sugars, and live on a diet that is virtually devoid of nutrients and still expect to shine.

I live in the same real world as you, so I want to

---

1   The word "diet" used throughout this book does not refer to a restricted diet, based on deprivation. Instead, it is used to refer to the way a person habitually eats.

enhance people's nutritional intake in a way that is practical for them. Let's say you eat 35 times a week, made up of three main meals and two snacks each day. And let's say that currently seven of those 35 meals meet my criteria for a health-enhancing, nutrient-dense meal. Well, if you simply add one real food meal or snack or smoothie each week for the next two months, your real food intake will then be at 15 out of your 35 meals, and you will have more than doubled the amount of nutrients going in, in eight tiny weeks out of your very long life! Plus seven fewer meals will now contain ingredients that have the potential to take away from your health and your shine. For most of you, this shift will feel simple, and it will also be delicious and health-enhancing! Unless a complete overhaul of your pantry, and essentially your life, appeals to you (and if it does — go for it!), gradual changes will be far more sustainable for you and/or your family.

When you begin to focus on taking great care of your physical health, a huge part of that involves taking good care of the way you feed yourself. It is difficult to be kind, compassionate, and patient with others, as well as yourself, when you are filling yourself with stimulants and food that contains very little, if any, nutritional value. Think about that. As Hippocrates so perfectly suggested:

> *Let food be thy medicine and*
> *medicine be thy food.*

A real food approach to eating:

✓ allows you to simply and easily increase the nutrient content of your diet through a high-plant diet

✓ supports optimal blood pH via a focus on increasing the green vegetable content of meals

✓ decreases the synthetic chemical load being consumed by encouraging the use of organic food

✓ enhances and supports detoxification processes through omitting liver loaders and supplying the nutrients necessary to optimize these functions

✓ supports the energy systems of the body through optimal nutrient intake while lowering the intake of substances that can interfere with the creation of energy.

Increasing Nutrient Content Through a High-Plant Diet

A health-enhancing diet is one based on plant foods. Incorporating more plant foods into your diet is the quickest and easiest way to increase nutrient density and hence your shine! Plant foods are good sources of soluble and insoluble fibre. Insoluble fibre helps provide bulk to our stools to keep our bowels regular, and is used to help feed our gut bacteria. Feeding the good bacteria is an essential component of keeping the balance between the good and not-so-good bacteria in the gut. A healthy digestive system is the foundation of great health and beautiful skin, as discussed in more detail in the digestion chapter. It is all very well to be consuming a nutrient-dense diet, but if your digestive system is not absorbing and utilizing these vitamins and minerals you will not reap the benefits.

Nutritionally, leafy greens are superstars. They not only contain vitamins and minerals, but they enhance the quality of your blood. Leafy green vegetables also contain amino acids, which are the building blocks of proteins. In your body, amino acids make up the cells of your immune system that help defend you from infections and cancer; they create the neurotransmitters that influence your mood, and they build the muscles that drive your metabolic rate and give you physical strength. The power of greens is well demonstrated by the way gorillas live, and, given that they are similar to humans from a DNA perspective but have not been influenced by marketing, we can learn a lot from their innate food choices. The diet of gorillas is over 50 per cent piths, shoots, and green leaves, and yet they have one of the highest muscle masses of any living creature. They eat some animal protein, which they obtain mostly from insects, but the ratio of greens to animals is enormously in favour of a high-plant diet.

Our bodies thrive on being supplied with living foods, so the more plants we incorporate into our diet, the better we feel. One of the main reasons plants accumulate nutrients is to develop future seeds so they can reproduce and the species can survive. Seeds require a high density of nutrients to fulfil their reproductive functions. Even once they have germinated they need a significant amount of energy and nutrition to sprout and survive. Sprouts are nutrient-packed powerhouses!

Plants accumulate nutrients long before they create their seeds, and there is no better place for accumulating and storing nutrients than in the leaves. Hence, greens leaves are one of the most nutritious foods on Earth. Seeds, too, are rich in nutrients, but plants don't want their offspring to be eaten, so many plants also add protective mechanisms to their seeds by endowing them with a range of inhibitors, alkaloids, and other substances that may be harmful to predators. Nature is truly amazing.

If you grow greens or herbs yourself, the best time to harvest them is before the formation of seeds. This is when the green leaves have the highest concentration of nutrients. After a plant blossoms, nutrients begin to accumulate inside the seeds, and once the seeds are gone there is almost no nutrition left in the leaves. They tend to turn yellow and dry out and fall off — think of a parsley plant after it has gone to seed — so that the remaining nutrients return to the soil and the plant can rest until the next growing season. Seasons and cycles in Nature all serve a purpose, and human health relies on these cycles to nourish and sustain our life.

SUPPORTING OPTIMAL BLOOD PH

The pH of your blood is always alkaline. It is crucial that you understand how this relates to your health before we go any further, so what follows is a quick refresher on pH from high-school chemistry.

The acidity or alkalinity of any solution is determined by how much hydrogen (H^+) and hydroxide (OH^-) ions are within the substance, and this is expressed as pH, meaning "power of hydrogen" (or "potential of hydrogen"). The pH of a solution is a mathematical calculation based on a scale from 0 to 14, where 7 is neutral. The theoretical pH of distilled water is 7, where the relative concentrations of H^+ and OH^- are equal. For every unit *below* pH 7, the concentration of H^+ increases by a factor of 10. Those kinds of solutions are *acidic*. For every unit *above* 7, the concentration of OH^- is increased similarly. Those kinds of solutions are *alkaline*.

Your blood is always alkaline. It is held within a very narrow range, with 7.365 being ideal, and your body will work very hard to keep you here. The foods and liquids you consume every day have a significant effect on the pH of your blood. Most high-water vegetables and some fruits, including lemons, have an alkaline effect on blood pH, while meat, dairy, and most grains are more acid-yielding.

A lemon, though acidic itself, will actually reduce the body's acidic load once its mineral contents are absorbed into the blood. This is because the predominant minerals within the lemon (for the science-minded among you, these are the electrically positive cations of calcium, potassium, sodium, and magnesium) have an alkalizing (acid-reducing) effect on blood chemistry. They do this by forming mineral hydroxides and carbonates in our cells, which act like molecular sponges to "soak up" excess acidity.

There is much debate about the diets of our ancient human ancestors and the precise ratio of animal to vegetable matter they consumed. What *is* known is that for outstanding health, the effect of animal food on blood chemistry, if it is eaten, must be buffered by a higher quantity of plant foods that will push blood chemistry to the more alkaline end of the spectrum. That way our blood is happy and our health can be optimal.

What we also know is that, since the Industrial Revolution began around 180 years ago, most people's diets have become more heavily dependent on foods that push our blood chemistry to the acidic end of the spectrum, and our bodies have not been able to adapt. The Industrial Revolution didn't just mean the beginning of railways and sewing machines, but also the introduction of processes for canning, refining sugars, and milling flour, all of which led to an unprecedented shift in the human diet. As people began to eat in this "progressive" way, choosing more and more "convenience" foods, they significantly reduced their intake of whole foods, particularly green vegetables, replacing them with more white flour and white sugar than had ever been consumed before throughout all of human history. When the human diet is based on highly-processed foods that are virtually devoid of all nutrients, health suffers.

Yet, I am often asked, given that people tend to be living longer these days in the Western world, if our diet is in general so lousy, why is longevity increasing? I answer this question with another question: Are we living too short and dying too long? It is quality of life that I care about so passionately. Now and always, you do not want to lose your independence and have to rely on another person to tie your shoelaces because you can no longer reach them because you are stiff or your tummy is so large you can't reach over it. You don't want to have to go to the hospital every other day to be hooked up to a dialysis machine because your kidneys can no longer clean your own blood. Yes, genes play a role. Of course they do. But, we need to remember that the health choices we make today influence the genes that will be switched on now, or down the track, as well as how we will feel and function both today and in the future.

Let that empower you to know that you can significantly decrease your risk of developing some of the major degenerative diseases in our world, along with positively influencing the quality of your life both today and in the future, simply by choosing a high-plant, nutrient-dense diet.

As mentioned above, it is critical that the pH of human blood stays as close as possible to 7.365 (slightly alkaline). If it drops below 7 (acidemia) or rises above 7.8 (alkalemia), coma and death can quickly follow. Consequently, the human body does everything in its power to ensure that the pH of its tissues remains within stringent confines.

For example, to preserve pH balance under conditions of chronic acid load (as occurs with diets high in processed foods and alcohol), the body must continually draw on its alkaline reserves by releasing calcium, potassium, and magnesium from the bone matrix to neutralize excess acid. In addition, the body begins to break down muscle protein in order to release the amino acid glutamine. In turn, glutamine is converted to glutamic acid (glutamate) by the liver and, in doing so, it binds with excess hydrogen ions and ammonia is generated. The ammonia is then excreted in the urine, along with chloride ions that are needed to balance the electrochemical charge.

If all of that sounds too scientific, all you need to know is that too many foods that push your blood to the acidic end of the spectrum will drive your body to release minerals that are alkaline in their nature from their storage houses, the bones, into the blood, in order to even out the effects of the acid. The blood is happy, but your bones have been thinned in the process. I personally believe this is one the major reasons why we see so much more osteoporosis in the West, compared with those eating a traditional Eastern diet, which is based mainly on plant foods, and little or no processed food.

Amp up your greens for outstanding bone health, as this way your body will not need to call on your bones to release their precious minerals to counterbalance the effects of an overly acidic lifestyle. Your muscles will also love you by preventing the progressive muscle wasting that can come from an overly acidic diet. Given that your muscles significantly influence your metabolic rate, your ability to utilize carbohydrates for energy, and your strength, they are worth maintaining or, preferably, building.

Blood pH is also believed to influence the body's ability to burn body fat or store it. The best way to imagine it is that every cell in the human body is bathed in blood (plasma), and when the pH is ever so slightly too acidic, the cells hold onto additional fat to insulate themselves from the "acid burn". So a way of eating that fosters alkalinity also serves your body's ability to burn body fat as a fuel.

In addition to facilitating the development of osteoporosis, and in some cases an increase in body fat, an acid-promoting diet initiates a broad cascade of biochemical and physiological changes to our chemistry that can damage our health and also our physical appearance.

This cascade includes chronic oxidative stress, enhanced catabolism (muscle wasting and destruction of skeletal reserves), elevation of insulin and cortisol (both linked to body fat storage and a host of other biochemical effects, as described in *Accidentally Overweight*), systemic inflammation, and impaired immunity. Each of these situations has its own documented adverse health effects — so just imagine the implications when they are all happening at the same time! These processes are essentially what science has come to call "aging", and yet you can already see that a high-plant, nutrient-dense diet plays a powerful role in counterbalancing these "aging" processes. Let it empower you to know that a high-plant diet can have a significant impact on the prevention of these undesirable biochemical states, and hence a wonderfully positive and powerful effect on your quality of life and the way you age.

The Difference Between Digestion Acidity and Blood Alkalinity

It can be confusing when you hear about the importance of acidity in the digestive system (which is discussed in the Beautiful Digestion chapter) and the importance of alkalinity in the blood. As mentioned in the digestion section ahead, having optimal acid levels in the stomach is essential for effective digestion, both in the stomach itself, plus to set up the pH gradient as the digestive tract continues. If the acid in the stomach is not acidic enough, the food will not be broken down correctly, and partially undigested food will end up too far along the digestive tract. If this occurs, that food is fermented, and this drives undesirable gut bacteria to take up residence in the colon. These bacteria often make lactic acid, which further impairs digestion, nutrient absorption, and liver function, as well as adding additional acid to the body's load. Poor digestion has an acidifying effect on blood chemistry, a significant reason why it is so important to optimize this process.

DECREASING THE SYNTHETIC CHEMICAL LOAD

Decreasing the synthetic chemical load is another important aim of optimal nourishment.

Food

Eating more organically or biodynamically grown food, or simply choosing spray-free options, can play a major role in achieving this. When it comes to pesticides, in my opinion we are guinea pigs when it comes to the effects of long-term consumption of these substances. The reason a conventionally grown apple looks so perfect is because it has been sprayed to make it look that way. We cannot see or taste the chemicals on its skin, but they are there. Pesticides have to be tested before they can be used on food for human consumption. However, they are often tested for such a relatively brief amount of time that I do not believe we can compare tests done over, say, a six-month period, to being exposed to these substances over an entire lifetime. What also cannot be tested is what happens when the chemicals are mixed, and they get mixed inside our body every day, when we eat conventionally grown produce.

Fresh food the way it comes in Nature is an incredibly important part of our diet. While I do not want to scare you off from eating a conventionally farmed apple, I do want to encourage you to choose organic produce whenever you can. Also think about the way you eat the food. We peel a banana. It may have been sprayed, but how much gets through the skin? We actually don't know. But surely there would be less chemical residue in the flesh of a banana than on the skin. So perhaps choosing a conventionally grown banana is not too bad. No one really knows yet. When it comes to an apple, though, we usually eat the whole fruit, so you would be better to choose an organic (or biodynamically grown) apple wherever possible.

What is biodynamic agriculture? It is the scientific use of crop rotation, composting, integrated soil, crop, and pest management, and animal husbandry pioneered in the early 20th century. These agricultural practices were later popularized by the organic movement. Both forms of agriculture are ecologically sound, and are fundamental to the health of the Earth, plants, and human beings. As Dr Rudolf Hauschka described, "biodynamic agriculture applies an organic and sustainable approach to farming that considers not only the health of the ecosystem but also the rhythms of the universe. The sun, moon, planets, and stars all influence how plants grow. It also applies herbal preparations to the earth to enliven and harmonise plants, compost, and soil, as well as addressing the source of problems rather than the symptoms. A biodynamic farmer looks to the ecosystem to find and correct the imbalance that caused (for example) an insect infestation."

Think about this. Organic food is the true cost of food. I once started and ran an organic café. Once a week, a local farmer delivered fresh greens picked that morning from his biodynamic farm. I always set aside some time on delivery days to chat with him, as he had wonderful tales to tell of life on his farm. One day, when I asked him how he was, his reply was along the lines of "not so good". When I enquired further, he went on to tell me that snails had invaded his broccoli patch, virtually overnight. When I paused to consider this, I realised that, if they took hold, a portion of this man's meagre livelihood would be lost. So I asked him how he deals with snails on his broccoli given that his farming principles do not involve spraying the patch to get rid of the invaders (which would have taken less than 30 minutes to do).

My farmer friend went on to tell me that snails lose

their "stick", their ability to suction onto things, in salty water. So he made up a bottle of salt and water, and he spent two days, crouched down on all fours, crawling between his broccoli plants, squirting saline water up under the fronds. Not only that, but he didn't kill the snails. Instead, he collected them in a bucket and fed them to the chickens, "to keep them in the food chain" as he so delightfully put it.

Consider each of these scenarios. Spray in under 30 minutes versus crawling around on your haunches for two days. For me, that illustrates precisely why organic and biodynamic food costs more. The price reflects the real cost of food, plus many foods grown this way have a greater nutritional value. The more of us who choose it, the cheaper it will become. Every time you spend money, you are casting a vote for the kind of world you want. The more we demand organic and say no to synthetic chemicals, the more organics will have to be supplied.

If organic food is simply not available in your area or it is too costly for you to buy, try this solution to remove pesticides. Pesticides tend to be fat-soluble, and general washing does not remove them. Washing food can remove dirt and germs, but not most pesticides. To wash food for both dirt and pesticides at the same time, fill your sink with three parts water to one part vinegar, and wash your fruits and vegetables. Then rinse them in fresh water, pat them dry, and store them for use. Do what is practical for you.

Plants have innate mechanisms designed to help protect themselves from pests. When a plant is left to grow of its own accord and is not sprayed with pesticides, the plant creates substances within itself to help ward off pests. These substances don't just have the ability to help protect the plant, however; they also often behave as antioxidants (explained in more detail later) when humans consume them. And if the plants are sprayed, they no longer have to (and don't) produce these substances that enhance human health and help slow down the aging process from the inside out. So eating organic food is not just about what you miss out on — pesticides — but also what you get — more antioxidants.

Pesticides typically have to be altered inside the body before they can be excreted. The liver is one organ involved in this process. The liver has to prioritise detoxification processes, and if there are more liver loaders present than available pathways for this to occur, the pesticides are usually stored in the fatty tissue of your body. Hence when any weight loss process is undertaken, liver support is of immense importance.

Skin Care

You can also decrease the synthetic chemical load in your life by considering what you put on your skin. You only have to think about how nicotine patches work to realise that your skin is a direct route to your blood supply, and that your detoxification systems will have additional work to do. There are some beautiful skin-care companies out there who create highly effective products that contain zero synthetic ingredients. In my ideal world you could eat your skin care! This concept is discussed in more detail in the "Beautiful Skin, Hair and Nails" chapter.

Oestrogens

On another note, some herbicides contain compounds that can mimic oestrogen in the human body, in both males and females of all ages. This is of great concern. For oestrogen or oestrogen-like compounds to exert their effects, they have to bind to oestrogen receptors, and when they do, the lovely, or not so lovely, effects of oestrogen are felt. Given that children today are exposed to herbicides for their entire lifetimes, it is likely that their exposure to oestrogen-like compounds in addition to what the body produces itself (mostly from puberty onwards) is contributing to the earlier age of menarche being reported across the Western world. Please pause and consider the ramifications of this.

Synthetic Load Reduction

Decrease your regular intake of synthetic chemicals by choosing organic produce or growing some of your own food, such as herbs, whenever you can. However, if this overwhelms you, then don't start here. Come to this when you are ready. In the meantime, focus on enhancing your detoxification processes, discussed below, to upregulate your body's ability to excrete these substances and really enhance your shine!

ENHANCING AND SUPPORTING DETOXIFICATION PROCESSES

Another reason to eat real food is to enhance the body's ability to detoxify itself. Detoxification is a process that is often misunderstood. It goes on inside of us, all day every day. We wouldn't be alive without it. However, the lifestyle choices we make influence how efficiently our body detoxifies.

The liver plays a major role in detoxification, which is essentially a transformation process. The body takes substances that if they were to accumulate would harm you, and changes them into substances that are less harmful so that you can excrete them.

Substances that influence detoxification processes include alcohol, caffeine, synthetic substances (including medications, pesticides, and ingredients in skin care), trans fats (damaged fats usually found in bought cakes and biscuits, muesli bars, and deep-fried food), and refined sugars. The liver also has to detoxify substances your body makes itself, such as oestrogen and cholesterol, which can have their own impact on inner health and outer beauty, as explored in greater detail in a later chapter.

When I am guiding people with what foods serve their health, one element that is firmly in my mind is minimizing (or, in some cases, eliminating) what

I call the "liver loaders", as this allows the body to pull stored toxins out of storage to be processed and excreted. This is of critical importance to amazing skin, which I will discuss in more detail later. Secondly, food is designed to supply the body with the nutrients necessary for the detoxification processes in the body to work efficiently. For example, the first stage of detoxification by the liver requires B vitamins for that process to occur. Our best food sources of B vitamins are whole grains, and yet many people have cut them out, or at least back, in this high-protein era we are currently living through. Many people feel better without grains (or with less or only specific types, for example gluten-free grains) in their diet, and I am by no means suggesting you suddenly go back and eat bucket-loads of grains to get your B vitamins if you feel better without them. All I want to point out is that, unknowingly, people can miss out on nutrients crucial to the inner workings of their body and their optimal health.

Choosing a wide variety of whole foods — and perhaps trying some gluten-free grains, if gluten-containing grains disrupt your digestive system — may assist these vital cleaning systems in your body. Eating real food also tends to help with regular bowel motions, and this, too, enhances detoxification processes, as the liver no longer has to pick up the shortfall of digestion. The liver loves, and is stimulated by, bitter foods, and there is no better way to stimulate the bitter taste buds than with green leafy vegies.

When I ask people how they are, these days I most often hear "exhausted", "stressed", "busy", "frantic", "broken", and "tired". I don't want this for you. I want you to feel amazing; I want you to feel energized, vital, and alive. That is beautiful! Without energy, it is difficult to make your own dreams come true and contribute to those around you. When we are exhausted, everything is more difficult. How do you wake up in the morning? Do you bounce out of bed, grateful that a new day has dawned that you are blessed to be part of? Or do you press the snooze button six times, wondering how on Earth it can be morning already? Mostly I hear the latter.

What is your energy like over the course of a day? Do you feel like your blood glucose is less like the even flow of a river, and more akin to a roller coaster, with dramatic highs and lows in your moods and also your energy levels? When you have a burst of energy, does your temper explode? Or are you someone who simply wishes you could spend the next year in bed? My point? Your energy levels significantly influence the quality of your life and your shine.

Food is designed to energize us in a lovely, even way. If what you have been eating makes you want to go to sleep, then it hasn't been serving you. Eating real food helps support the energy systems in your body.

The concept of photosynthesis may not be something you have considered since high school ... or maybe you are currently at high school and you don't feel too compelled to learn about it. Well, here's how it relates to your beauty. Photosynthesis is a process essential to life. Photosynthesis is a process used by plants, and other organisms, to convert the light energy captured from the sun into chemical energy that can be used to fuel the organism's activities. Diagrammatically it looks like this:

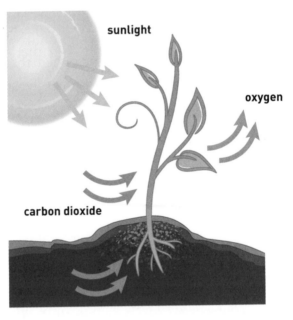

Green leaves are the only living things in the world that can transform sunshine into energy, creating a food that living creatures can consume. Hence, one of my favourite catch-phrases is "Amp up your greens — it's like eating sunshine."

Knowing this, it is hard to imagine how there could be life on Earth without greens. They produce chlorophyll, which, simply put, is liquid sunshine. Chlorophyll has powerful health properties of its own. In fact, haemoglobin, a component of human blood that helps transport oxygen around the body, is almost identical to chlorophyll.

All of the energy in food comes from the sun. Think about this every time you eat your greens, and amp up their proportion of your diet to enhance your energy systems and your sparkle.

The way energy is actually created within the body involves a series of biochemical pathways that nutrients drive. I had them pinned all over the walls of my bedroom while I was at university. I won't bore you by pinning them inside this book, although I am tempted to blow your mind at just how astonishing your body is, to show you the immense power of nutrients to drive your biochemistry and nourish you, and to remind you that life truly is miraculous! Just know that by increasing the nutrient density of your diet, you help enhance your energy systems, which can lead not only to a healthier life but a much happier one, too.

Flexitarian Eating

MEAT AND SEAFOOD

Significantly increasing the plant content of your diet is a powerful way to boost nutrient density essential to great health, vitality, and shine. So what about meat and fish? Nutrition polarizes people. We all eat, and therefore we all have our own opinions about what consists of a healthy diet. I always encourage people to eat in a way that nourishes *their* body, mind, and soul, and for some this means following a vegetarian or vegan diet.

However, many people choose to eat meat and/or fish, and describe feeling more nourished when they include it in their diet. My message to you is simple: eat the real food that nourishes *you*. Be rigid with your eating if, and only if, that serves you and/or the planet, depending on your beliefs. For example, if you feel deep in your heart that living a vegan lifestyle is right for you, then be true to that. Be sure, however, that you are getting optimum amounts of vitamin B_{12}, iron, and zinc, in particular.

A concept I would love to introduce you to, though, is what I call having a "flexitarian" approach to eating. I want to guide you to be in touch with what your *body* needs, not what your head tells you you want, or what a rule you created for yourself, possibly years ago, dictates, if this rule no longer serves you or the planet. A flexible approach enables you to nourish your body with what it needs, when it needs it. For example, there will be days when you feel that a meal that includes rice will nourish you beautifully, whereas there may be other days when you feel that rice won't serve you; you may feel like you will feel tired after eating it. But if you have a rule that says, for example, carbs after 3pm are bad, then you won't eat rice for dinner, no matter how much your body needs what rice offers. I find people also define themselves using how they eat as a descriptive: "I'm a vegetarian", for example. And I have met countless people who judge others for how they choose to eat, but judgement does not serve your health, or the planet, or anyone you meet. Eat in a way that feels right for you, and allow others to do the same.

If you eat meat, opt for grass-fed, free-range, or preferably organic. I appreciate that these options may cost more economically. However, in my opinion and based on my observation of people's diets over the past 15 years, many people would benefit from reducing their portion sizes of meat. Choose good-quality cuts of meat, and serve approximately a fist-sized portion for a main meal. Organic lamb, for example, provides protein, B group vitamins including B_1, B_2, B_3, B_6, and B_{12}, as well as the minerals iron and zinc in highly bioavailable forms, which means the body is able to utilize the minerals easily.

When it comes to seafood we experience a great divide in opinions again. Understandably, there is reason for concern about including seafood in your diet, as more information is emerging about heavy-metal contamination. Reducing your exposure to mercury is essential. If you eat fish, it is best to choose small, white fish, which have a lower risk of mercury contamination. Small fish are a better choice because they have had less exposure and time to accumulate mercury. However, remember that having good zinc levels in your body is critical for your body to be able to detoxify and excrete any heavy metals that you are exposed to, such as through air pollution from cars.

Fish is an example of a nutrient-dense food. Besides containing protein and nutrients such as selenium and vitamin D, fish also contains the anti-inflammatory omega-3 fatty acids. Clinically, omega-3 fatty acids have been shown to reduce the risk of developing many degenerative diseases, including heart disease. For pregnant women, breastfeeding mothers, and women of childbearing age, fish can supply the body with **DHA,** an omega-3 fatty acid that is beneficial for brain development. Flaxseeds (linseeds) are high in another omega-3 fatty acid known as EPA. The human body can convert EPA into DHA, a process that is upregulated during pregnancy. Again, I encourage you to eat what nourishes you. Just be sure to include some omega-3-rich foods.

If you eat chicken, purchasing organic chicken is highly recommended. Organically-grown chickens have been fed an organically-grown diet and have been raised without the use of antibiotics, and free-range chickens have been allowed access to the outdoors as opposed to being confined to the henhouse, with some producers also feeding them an organic diet. Chicken is a good source of protein and also contains niacin (vitamin B$_3$), which helps the body convert food into fuel (energy). Additionally, niacin is involved in the production of sex and stress hormones in the adrenal glands, critical processes for inner and outer health, which you'll learn more about in later chapters. It also contains methionine, an amino acid involved in mood regulation and the maintenance of our DNA.

If yours has been a "meat with every meal" household up until now, consider starting "meatless Mondays", and eat only plant-based foods that day. Once you and/or family members/housemates experience the taste sensation of a vegetable-based meal you like (try some from the *Real Food Chef* cookbook!), you may find that three vegetarian meals per week becomes an easy option. Keep in mind, too, the recommendations from the most respected source of cancer prevention research and information, the World Cancer Research Fund (WCRF), which state, "limit your intake of red meat to no more than 300 grams per week, and avoid processed meat". Don't go meatless if it is not your thing and if meat nourishes you, which it does for many. Just eat plenty more vegetables and other plant foods than meat.

FATS

Nutrition information tends to move in cycles. Whether the current focus is on decreasing carbohydrates or increasing protein, one thing seems to remain constant: many people have a fear of fat.

Yet, so much can go wrong with our health and our beauty if we eat too little fat. Your skin can dry out without enough!

What is commonly misunderstood is the essential role that fats play in our body and especially in our beauty. Not all fat is created equal, though. Fats are composed of building blocks called fatty acids, just as proteins are comprised of their building blocks, amino acids.

There are three major categories of fatty acids: saturated, polyunsaturated, and monounsaturated. Of concern more recently is the generation of trans fats, which are found mainly in processed foods, specifically deep-fried foods, bought cakes and biscuits, and muesli bars. Some research suggests that the *type* of fat you eat is actually more important than the total amount. Depending on the current state of your diet, I often encourage people to consume more fats, particularly from whole food sources. Consuming adequate fat, and the right fats, helps you manage your mood, stay alert, and regulate blood sugar; it even assists with weight management.

Fats are also needed to help absorb vitamins such as A D, E, and K, as well as to maintain healthy skin, as explored in more detail in the Beautiful Nutrients chapter. They are an integral part of our immunity and brain development. Fat is also our most concentrated source of energy, and helps to keep us warm and protect our organs. The Mediterranean diet, high in monounsaturated fats, is linked with low blood pressure and lower incidences of heart disease.

By choosing real food, you will naturally avoid poor-quality fats such as trans fats. If you experience sweet cravings in the afternoon, add more fat to your meals, particularly at lunch (and even more so if it was very low in fat), in the form of avocado, coconut, nuts, seeds, organic butter, tahini, or oily fish, and observe if your desire for sweet foods mid-afternoon diminishes. Many people have become scared of using oils and nuts due to their high-energy (calorie) content, but good fats actually slow down the release of glucose into your blood stream, requiring less insulin (a fat storage hormone discussed at length in my book *Accidentally Overweight*), and allowing you to stay full for longer.

Fats in a Nutshell ...

Fats are a vital component of the human diet. There are numerous types of fats, some of which are essential for survival. This means that the body cannot synthesize them and that they must be eaten.

The different types of fats are:

- **saturated,** such as those found in coconut

- **monounsaturated,** such as those found in olives, avocadoes, and macadamia nuts, as well as the oils from these foods

- **polyunsaturated,** of which there are two types:

- omega-6, such as those found predominantly in certain nuts and seeds, and oils from these foods

- omega-3, such as those found in oily fish, linseeds (flaxseeds), walnuts, and pecans, and oils from these foods.

The above fats all play crucial roles in obtaining and maintaining optimal health. They help our immune system defend us from infection and cancer, and they help create our sex hormones, which are vital for fertility, happiness, and the appearance of our skin — just to name a few effects! Importantly, they also help mediate inflammation, which is one of the ways we age from the inside out. The list of benefits is almost endless.

You have to eat fat to burn fat, and I have met thousands of people who eat too little fat. If you eliminate fat or eat too small an amount, your body tends to believe that there is some sort of famine going on, and it stores body fat, thinking it is doing you a big favour by helping you get through this period of supposed restriction.

Include fat from whole food sources. Such foods add to the satiety factor of each meal, as well as to the nutritional content. For the body to be able to extract fat-soluble vitamins from food, for example, they must be in the presence of fat. So often I am asked: "How much avocado can I eat?" When you start to eat more real food meals, you will be able to answer that question yourself! Your body is your best guide, and I want you to be in touch with its signals rather than having them masked by a diet full of processed fats, and refined sugars and flours. There will be days when half an avocado will serve you at lunchtime, while on other days only a whole one will do. You might begin to notice that when avocado is in the presence of lemon juice and herbs it tastes even better, and taste may be one of the aspects you need in your food for it to be satisfying.

Choose fat from real food sources. Your skin, your hair, and your eyes — just to name a few beauty spots! — will love you for it.

Before we explore specific foods and the wonderful impact they can have on your beauty, it is important at this stage in your journey through this book that you understand a few key concepts about the physical way in which we age, including the way wrinkles are formed.

How Real Food Slows the Aging Process

Physically, two processes rapidly drive the aging process, and they are also linked to many modern-day illnesses, including heart disease, type 2 diabetes, cancer, and Alzheimer's disease. The two processes are *oxidation* and *inflammation*.

Oxidation is one way we age, and an enormous aspect of the *Beauty from the Inside Out* concept is guiding you to prevent or certainly limit the damage done by oxidation. It has significant inner health and outer beauty consequences. Oxidative damage is done by substances known as free radicals, which are single oxygen molecules that can hurt your tissues and other vital substances in your body.

Humans stay alive through a process called respiration, meaning that we breathe in oxygen, and we exhale carbon dioxide. If you could see oxygen in space, it is two 'O's (two oxygen molecules) stuck together. The diagram below illustrates what I am about to describe.

$$O_2$$

$$O = O$$

$$O^- \text{ (free radical)}$$

$$A/O \text{ (antioxidant/donator)}$$

$$O = O$$

$$O_2$$

Free radical protection from antioxidants: The oxygen donation of antioxidants.

When we breathe, oxygen splits apart, forming two

single oxygen molecules — free radicals — and they are angry little critters, as they have lost their buddy and are now able to damage your tissues. Free radicals do have minimal benefit within the body, which includes assisting white blood cells to reduce infection. However, the number of free radicals within the blood is greatly increased by stress, high-intensity exercise, cigarette smoke, and pollutants such as pesticides and heavy metals. You can see how modern-day living can mean that the number of free radicals in the body becomes high and stops serving our health, and begins to cause harm.

One of the major ways the body defends itself from free radical damage is through the consumption of antioxidants. Antioxidant-rich foods are our coloured plant foods. If you could imagine a large platter covered in beautiful, brightly coloured fresh produce, that platter would pack a massive antioxidant punch! The way it works is that the antioxidant donates one of its oxygen molecules back to the single guy (free radical) and they pair up. The oxygen is then as happy as a duck in water, and will no longer damage your tissues. Isn't that magical? And this is an enormous reason why people like me bark on and on about the immense importance of amping up the plant food content of your diet.

Oxidation is explored in detail in the Beautiful Detox chapter, but to thoroughly link this process to skin, I offer you this explanation. Your immune system is designed to protect you from infection and to play a role in dampening down inflammation. Immune cells will attack any substance that shows up in your body that they decide is foreign or poisonous, or that they believe you are better off without. These substances may appear in your food, water, or as viruses or bacteria that you ingest, which then generate free radicals (also known as oxidants). As you now understand, free radicals are highly reactive molecules, and they destroy cells and tissues by causing them to age, form scar tissue, and die. Free radicals cause all living things to age and decay. They are the reason an apple left on your bench turns brown and shrivels up.

In your skin, free radicals cause the moist collagen fibres that form its super-structure to become dry and shrivelled. When the foundation of your skin shrinks, the surface folds over on itself, forming wrinkles. The more free radicals in your system, the more your collagen shrinks, and the more wrinkles appear on your skin.

Free radicals also cause the inside of your arteries to become a landscape of lesions and sticky cholesterol plaques, described in detail in the Beautiful Detox chapter, which can eventually lead to a heart attack or stroke.

One of the most powerful ways to significantly impact your health and your appearance is to control the amount of oxidation and inflammation in your tissues. And the best ways to do this are to decrease the quantity of pollutants you are exposed to and increase the plant content of your diet. There are additional free articles about the power of anti-oxidants, as well as free recipes available at: www. drlibby.com/bioresources

INFLAMMATION

Inflammation is the other major way we age. Put simply, inflammation is your immune system's response to any problematic substance that has entered your body. How do things enter? You can ingest them, breathe them, or you can absorb them through your skin.

When your immune system perceives that a threatening substance is in your diet, for example, it mounts a powerful and multi-pronged attack on the "invader". Part of that response is to create inflammation, which we recognize as heat, swelling, and redness. This occurs wherever the immune system is engaged in a battle — in the tissues of your face, in your arteries, and/or in your vital organs, for example. Inflammation is essential to keeping us alive, but it also causes collateral damage, such as scarring and wrinkling.

The more pollutants we are exposed to, the more inflammation our body experiences, and the more rapidly we age.

"Beauty Foods"

When it comes to real food, for me they are all super foods. Each food has its own unique combination of nutritional value to offer you and your glow. Here is a list to show you some of the beauty benefits.

ALMONDS

A good source of vitamin E, copper, magnesium, manganese, potassium, calcium, and iron, all of which are essential to skin oxygenation and function.

APPLE CIDER VINEGAR

Helps stimulate digestion and may improve extraction of minerals and vitamins from your diet. It may also be a helpful natural remedy for dandruff, because the acids in the vinegar stop the fungus-causing chemical imbalances in the skin of the scalp.

ARTICHOKES

Regular consumption of these woody, fibrous vegetables is linked to healthier skin, and, in particular, improved skin luminosity.

AVOCADOS

A good source of biotin and monounsaturated fats, avocados help to prevent dry skin and brittle hair and nails; when applied topically, they help to hydrate dry skin. For me, they are a super special beauty food.

BEANS

Beans are a wonderful vegetarian source of protein. Protein breaks down into amino acids, which help speed the repair and regeneration of skin cells and collagen.

BEETROOTS

Beetroot contains nitrates, which produce a gas called nitric oxide in the blood, which widens blood vessels and lowers blood pressure; it is also important for blood flow to skin.

BLUEBERRIES

One of the richest sources of antioxidants, these beautiful and delicious berries counteract premature aging.

BRAZIL NUTS

These are a good source of the antioxidant selenium, which helps increase the number of infection-fighting white blood cells in the body, as well as protect against cellular damage. For skin care, selenium's antioxidant properties regenerate vitamins E and C, thereby decreasing the aging of skin. A truly amazing nut!

BROCCOLI AND CAULIFLOWER

Vegetables worthy of their superstar accolades, they are potent sources of antioxidants, as well as many vitamins and minerals, which help aid cellular repair. Vegetables in the *Brassica* family contain indoles, substances that help the liver detoxify hormones, which can help with sex hormone balance, which is critical for clear skin.

COCONUTS

Coconuts are great for your skin and body, inside and out. Containing vitamins A and C, calcium, iron, and natural proteins, coconuts also contain medium-chain triglycerides, which are a wonderful fuel for the body, and also possess antibacterial properties. Lauric acid, for example, has been scientifically shown to have a stronger action against the bacteria often involved with acne than benzoyl peroxide, an ingredient in many medicated skin washes and some prescription acne medications. Topically, coconut oil is a great way to moisturize and cleanse your skin naturally.

CUCUMBERS

The high water content means it is a very hydrating choice, and is a wonderful way to reduce swelling or puffiness around eyes.

EGGS

Eggs are a complete source of protein. They contain biotin, an essential vitamin that protects against dry skin, and is also helpful for nail and hair health.

Eggs also contain iron, which is vital for oxygenation of the entire body, including the skin.

FIGS

Figs keep your digestive tract moving, which is critical for elimination pathways and the clarity of your skin. They contain calcium, an important mineral that allows the body to relax — and by the end of this book, you will understand how crucial activating the rest and repair mechanisms of the body is for inner health and outer beauty.

FRESH OILY FISH

This is a wonderful source of omega-3, which dampens down inflammation in the body and also helps keep skin moisturised. Fresh salmon also contains astaxanthin, a carotenoid that improves skin elasticity.

GREEN TEA

This wonderful skin-friendly beverage is packed full of antioxidants that are protective against cellular damage throughout the body, including the aging process of the skin.

KALE

Kale is an excellent source of the beauty vitamins A, C, and E, which have potent anti-aging properties and help promote healthy new cell growth. It is also loaded with minerals, such as magnesium and calcium, which healthy skin needs; these minerals are also critical to our ability to relax and are highly alkaline.

KIWIFRUIT

Kiwifruit is a rich source of vitamin C and antioxidants, which help keep skin firm and slow down the formation of wrinkles, and are also great for healthy teeth and bones. The antioxidants in kiwifruit have also been shown to help protect against cancer and heart disease.

LEMONS

Rich in vitamin C, lemons are great for the skin and also stimulate digestion — starting your day with lemon in warm water is a wonderful way to kick-start your digestion. The goodies in lemons are crucial for all aspects of beauty, obtaining the maximum nutrition from your diet and helping to supply your skin, hair and nails with nutrients.

NETTLE TEA

Nettle tea has an anti-inflammatory effect, and helps calm the skin and improve conditions like eczema and acne. It is extremely detoxifying, thanks to high levels of antioxidants.

OLIVE OIL

High-quality olive oil is a good source of mono-unsaturated fats, which offer protective benefits for heart health. It contains fatty acids that help keep skin soft and supple, and used in hair treatments, skin care, and lip balms, it helps restore shine and vitality.

ORGANIC BUTTER

This is a source of a wide variety of vitamins and minerals which are beneficial for skin, bone, and nervous system health. Organic butter is another good source of lauric acid, with its powerful antibacterial and antifungal actions.

PARSLEY

Its flavonoids, especially luteolin, have been shown to function as antioxidants that combine with highly reactive oxygen-containing molecules and help prevent oxygen-based damage to cells. Parsley has anti-inflammatory properties, is highly alkaline, and contains vitamin C and iron, important for the oxygenation of every tissue in your body. One of my absolute favourite foods.

PEPPERMINT TEA

Known for its potent healing and calming properties, peppermint tea is a wonderful skin-supporting change from normal tea that also supports digestion.

POMEGRANATES

Pomegranates are a rich source of vitamin C. They also help collagen production and increase the skin's capacity to heal when consumed.

SPINACH

This leafy green vegetable is rich in a wide range of nutrients and antioxidants. It is loaded with lutein, which keeps your vision and your eyes healthy and sparkling.

SPROUTS

A wonderful nutrient boost sprinkled on salads or soups, sprouts are packed full of minerals, including calcium, magnesium, manganese, and phosphorus, all of which support healthy, clear, and glowing skin.

SUNFLOWER SEEDS

Sunflower seeds are a good source of vitamin E, a protective antioxidant that helps skin glow. They also contain zinc, which keeps your skin, hair, and eyes healthy, and is critical for wound healing and scar prevention.

SWEET POTATOES

Sweet potatoes contain beta-carotene, a powerful antioxidant that helps slow the aging process.

TOMATOES

This great source of the antioxidant lycopene is considered a high-carotenoid fruit — both of these nutrients have been shown to slow down cellular damage from free radicals.

WALNUTS

Walnuts are a rich source of omega-3 fats, which help put shine in your hair and aid in making skin smooth and soft.

WATERCRESS

Leafy greens that are jammed full of antioxidants, as well as the minerals manganese, carotene, and potassium, watercress has a high water content, which assists with hydration.

Eating more, not less — eating real

The heart of my food message for supporting inner health and outer beauty is not about focusing on eating less of anything. I want to encourage you to focus on eating more — more real food, and mostly plants. If you struggle to eat less refined sugar, for example, eating more greens can help curb your desire for sweet food, since the bitter nature of the greens helps shift your preferences.

I would love to hear about your experience with this on my website or on social media, as your story can inspire and support others. One of the ways you show that you care about yourself is through the way you feed yourself. Nourish yourself with a real food focus.

The best and most beautiful things in the world cannot be seen or even touched ~ they must be felt with the heart.

Helen Keller

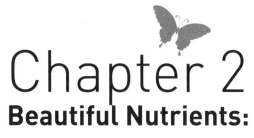

Chapter 2
Beautiful Nutrients:
essential factors for your beauty

From the soil, health and beauty are born. The soil contains minerals, such as calcium and magnesium, which we need to live. But we can't eat the soil, so we need a medium that is able to supply us with the earth's nutrients. The middlemen are plants, as they absorb the nutrients from the soil and make them available to us as food. Isn't that an incredible way to think about how we obtain the nutrients that sustain our life?

However, if the soil is deficient in nutrients, then those nutrients are not in the food. So the quality of the soil where our food is grown plays an enormous role in our health and beauty.

Nutrients

You have probably noticed that certain nutrients appear in skin care for topical application. I am a fan, however, of supplying all of the cells of the body with nutrients so that they can be distributed where they need to go, including nourishing your skin.

Let's take a look at the key nutrients involved with outward shine. Firstly, we will explore the role of the fat-soluble vitamins, vitamins A, D, E, and K, and, secondly, the water-soluble vitamins, which are all of the B-group vitamins and vitamin C. And, thirdly, we will look at some phytochemicals, fatty acids, and other substances that play a role in beauty mechanisms, substances all naturally occurring in plants. You will notice that some nutrients have a more detailed explanation about their involvement in your shine, while others are briefer. All vitamins and minerals are critical for your inner health and outer beauty, but some mechanisms of action require more explanation!

Fat-soluble vitamins

VITAMIN A

Vitamin A is often associated with healthy vision, but it is also essential for healthy, vibrant, glowing skin. Synthetically-derived retinoids (forms of vitamin A) have been used as treatments for severe acne and psoriasis since the 1980s, not to mention the countless formulas cosmetic companies sell containing vitamin A to support aging or troublesome skin. Vitamin A influences the physiology of the skin in a number of ways. When it comes to acne or blackheads, it acts to inhibit sebaceous gland activity. Regulating sebaceous glands is the aim of a lot of cosmetic solutions for the skin, as glandular activity determines if your skin is "oily", via the production of sebum. Vitamin A promotes cell turnover in the skin, and also thickens and stimulates the dermis — where your collagen, elastin, and blood vessels are — which increases blood flow to the surface of the skin and can lessen the appearance of wrinkles. Vitamin A actually increases the deposition of collagen and slows the breakdown of your collagen and elastin.

The term "vitamin A" makes it sound like there is just one vitamin called "vitamin A", but that is not the case. Vitamin A actually covers a broad group of related nutrients, each of which provide unique health benefits. To simplify the concept, we can divide vitamin A into two categories: retinoids and carotenoids. Retinoid forms of vitamin A are of particular importance for night vision, maintaining normal vision, fighting infections, for red blood cell production, and also for pregnancy. During gestation, retinoids contribute to the baby's embryonic growth, including the development of the heart, lungs, kidneys, eyes, and bones, and the circulatory, respiratory, and central nervous systems. They are also particularly important for women who are about to give birth, because they help with postpartum tissue repair.

Carotenoids also provide unique health benefits. Most carotenoids function as antioxidants and have anti-inflammatory effects, two of the processes that are key in slowing the aging process from the inside out. Two of the better-known carotenoids are lutein and zeaxanthin. Similar to retinoids, both of these carotenoids are essential to vision and are associated with the prevention of age-related macular degeneration. Some carotenoid (plant forms) of vitamin A can effectively be converted into retinoid forms in some individuals. Many different factors influence whether you are able to convert carotenoids forms into retinoid forms. Digestive system problems, excessive use of alcohol, exposure to toxic chemicals, or an imbalanced vitamin A to D ratio — as a result of high-dose supplementation and/or medications — can all interfere with the body's ability to make this conversion. Beta-carotene — found in carrots, pumpkins, sweet potatoes, and spinach — has the best conversion ratio to retinoids. For vegetarians and vegans, it is important to note that research indicates that you can obtain adequate vitamin A by incorporating different plant sources of vitamin A. Allowing the body to control the degree of conversion tends to provide the best regulation of both carotenoid and retinoid levels

Lack of vitamin A can cause the skin to become scaly, and it also stops mucous secretions, which can result in dry eyes. Rough, dry skin can be a sign of vitamin A deficiency, which can appear as rough, raised bumps on the back of the arms. This condition is clinically referred to as keratosis pilaris, and is thought to affect up to 40 per cent of the population. Some of the most commonly prescribed medications for skin conditions such as acne, eczema, and psoriasis are derived from vitamin A (retinol). The active ingredients in the drugs used to treat skin conditions utilise the same methods of action as vitamin A derived from natural sources. It is important not to assume that foods rich in vitamin A have the same effect as synthetically-derived medications, but eating a variety of foods that contain vitamin A will support and improve many skin conditions. The power of a real food, high plant-based diet can be game-changing when it comes to your skin.

The most vitamin A-rich foods are liver and cod-liver oil, but other sources include kidneys, organic butter from pastured (grass-fed) cows, and egg yolks. Vegetarian sources of vitamin A include leafy green vegetables, orange and yellow vegetables, tomatoes, and certain fruits, such as apricots and grapefruit. Toxicity from food is very rare; when it does occur, it is usually due to the excess consumption of liver. Carotenoids are fat-soluble, so adequate fat at the time of consumption is necessary for optimal absorption. To tackle this practically, when you eat a vegetarian source of Vitamin A, such as carrots, pair it with tahini, nut butter, organic butter, or avocado to improve absorption.

Isotretinoin

For the treatment of acne, the most-prescribed retinoid drug is 13-cis-retinoic acid (isotretinoin). Notice the name, even though it is a big, long scientific word? Notice the "retinoic acid" part of the name? That means it is vitamin A-based. This man-made vitamin A-based drug is designed to reduce the size and secretion of the sebaceous glands and reduce bacterial numbers in both the ducts and the skin surface. It appears to work by reducing sebum production, which can act as a nutrient source for bacteria. It is also designed to decrease inflammation. All of these changes are only temporary, however, and are related to the dose and duration of treatment with the drug.

Isotretinoin is also, unfortunately, a teratogen with a number of potential side effects. A teratogen is an agent, such as a drug, virus, or radiation, which causes malformation of an embryo or foetus. Studies have also shown a link between the use of this substance and depressive symptoms. Consequently, its use requires strict medical supervision.

I share this in-depth information about vitamin A and the way it works in the body to show you just one example of a drug based on (not the same as) a nutrient. However, this doesn't get to the heart of *why* someone's body can't regulate this system at a particular stage in life. Dietary change can go a long way to making an enormous difference in someone's skin. I have witnessed it hundreds of times. Sometimes the immune system and/or sex hormone balance need support as well, and this, coupled with dietary change, will improve their skin. There is always a reason why someone's skin is a challenge; we just need to find it for that individual. I will explore this in greater detail in the Beautiful Skin chapter.

Vitamin A in a Nutshell

- There are two basic forms of vitamin A (retinoids and carotenoids), and both forms provide unique health benefits. Retinoid forms are derived from animal sources, whereas carotenoids are derived from plants.

- If you are a vegetarian/vegan, your body is able to convert carotenoids into retinoids. You don't have to eat animal foods to obtain retinoid forms of vitamin A. However, it is possible for this conversion to be compromised.

- Many factors can compromise the body's ability to convert carotenoids into retinoids, including digestive problems, gut dysbiosis, excessive alcohol consumption, excessive exposure to toxins, imbalanced intake of vitamin A and vitamin D in supplement form, and medications.

- Some vitamin A health benefits require you to eat foods that are rich in specific carotenoids. A great example is eye health and the unique role of the carotenoids lutein and zeaxanthin in the health of our eyes. Lutein and zeaxanthin are found in green leafy vegetables and egg yolks.

- As carotenoids are fat-soluble, adequate fat in the diet is essential. When you consume carotenoids sources of vitamin A, make sure you pair it with a source of fat such as nuts, seeds, oily fish, avocado, organic butter or tahini.

VITAMIN D

It often amazes people to learn that the body, via the skin, has the ability to manufacture as much as 10,000 IU of vitamin D after 20 to 30 minutes of summer sun exposure. Yet many people today are deficient and there is a host of reasons why, including not spending enough time outdoors. Here is how vitamin D becomes active and is able to do its magical work toward your health and beauty.

Vitamin D is not one chemical, but many, and a conversion process is required to generate active vitamin D. A type of cholesterol, 7-dehydrocholesterol, is present in the skin. The sun's ultraviolet B (UVB) rays convert the cholesterol into vitamin D_3. In contrast, most dietary supplements are manufactured by exposing a plant sterol to ultraviolet energy, thus producing vitamin D_2. Because their function is almost identical, D_2 and D_3 are lumped together under the name vitamin D, but neither functions until the liver and kidneys transform them into active vitamin D. This is diagrammatically represented below.

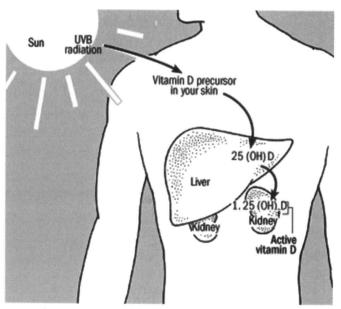

The creation of active vitamin D: Sunlight acts on the cholesterol in the skin, creating an inactive form of vitamin D for the liver and kidneys to activate.

One reason I believe so many people today are deficient in active vitamin D is because of what I call "liver congestion". When the liver is unable to keep up with its lifesaving work of detoxification, due to the regular overconsumption of liver loaders (explored in more detail in the Beautiful Detox chapter), I am concerned that other liver-related processes are impeded, this vitamin D conversion included. Taking better care of the liver may just make a vital difference to vitamin D status.

The active form of vitamin D_3 controls many processes essential to beauty, including skin repair and skin-cell production. Vitamin D is also critical for the health of the hair follicles, and hair loss has been associated with vitamin D deficiencies (among other nutrient deficiencies). Vitamin D is essential to bone health and the prevention of numerous degenerative diseases, including cancer. So be sure to get the vitamin D you need!

VITAMIN E

Vitamin E is a powerful antioxidant that can penetrate through layers of skin, assisting the body with the natural wound-healing process. Vitamin E also helps to renew skin cells, making them stronger by reducing oxidative stress. When the body experiences oxidative stress, cells can become weak, and your skin may look dull.

An optimal intake of vitamin E may also help reduce the appearance of wrinkles, and, when applied topically, vitamin E soothes dry or rough skin. Food sources of vitamin E include sunflower seeds, almonds, and avocados. Vitamin E deficiency signs include dry skin and poor wound healing.

As an aside, when I was a teenager, the Western world was bombarded with the message that fat was bad and that dietary intake of fats was to be kept to as low a level as possible for good health. Being the health-conscious girl I was, I did as I was told and pretty much cut fat out of my diet. My dear mum suggested on occasion that fat was actually very important for health and that I needed to include some from whole-food sources. But I thought the media knew better than Mum, until I stayed at a friend's house one night. Just before we went to bed, my friend asked her mum, who was rather cool, if we could have one of her vitamin E capsules, and she agreed. When I asked my friend what it was for, she said, "Mum says it prevents wrinkles." Yet, when I looked at the capsule, it looked just like oil. So I read the label and, sure enough, it was 100 per cent wheat-germ oil. On my return home to my dear mum, I told her about the vitamin E, and she explained that it is a fat-soluble vitamin only found in foods with fat in them. After years of Mum doing her best to get me to eat more fat, it took the vitamin E experience on my sleepover to convince me of the merits of fat. As science and my mum explain, without enough good fats, among other things, we dry out, and that's not a good look! So be sure to get plenty of whole-food sources of vitamin E in your diet. It is also a nutrient you can supplement to support your health and hence your beauty.

VITAMIN K

There are two main forms of vitamin K: phylloquinone (vitamin K_1), which is found in green leafy vegetables, such as broccoli and spinach; and vitamin K_2, the main storage form in animals, which also has a group of subtypes known as menaquinones. The K_2 forms can be synthesized from K_1 by microflora in the gut, and are also found in the diet in meat and fermented foods, such as sauerkraut.[2]

One of the health benefits of vitamin K not often discussed is its role in healthy skin. Research shows that people who cannot metabolize vitamin K end up with severe premature skin wrinkling. Adequate dietary vitamin K appears to prevent the hardening of our skin's elastin, the protein that gives skin the ability to spring back, which helps smooth out lines and wrinkles. Researchers believe that vitamin K deficiency is highly likely to be linked to wrinkling because vitamin K_2 (menaquinone) is necessary to

2   Those on blood-thinning medication need to consult their health-care professional before altering vitamin K intake.

stop calcium from depositing into elastin fibres. Optimal vitamin K levels are also believed to assist in the prevention of varicose veins.

Unlike the other fat-soluble vitamins (vitamins A, D, and E), vitamin K is not stored in the body, so it must be provided daily, and a real food way of eating is critical to getting the nutrient density necessary. So "amp up your greens"! Despite vitamin K_2's production by healthy intestinal bacteria, humans can develop a deficiency of the vitamin in as few as seven days on a vitamin K-deficient diet, a situation that is likely to occur even sooner if digestion is compromised.

Absorption of vitamin K, like that of other fat-soluble nutrients (A, D and E), depends on healthy liver, gallbladder, and digestive function. Deficiency is more likely in people with digestive problems like celiac disease or irritable bowel syndrome, or those who have had intestinal bypass surgery, since all increase the likelihood of fat malabsorption.

Water-soluble Vitamins

B-GROUP VITAMINS

B-group vitamins are essential to skin health. Vitamin B_1 (thiamine) is beneficial to hair and skin because it increases blood flow to the cells. Vitamin B_3 (niacinamide) and vitamin B_5 (pantothenic acid) are helpful in the process of skin regeneration, and can help slow the signs of aging skin when consumed daily in the diet. Synthetically-derived vitamin B_3 is becoming a very popular skin-care ingredient due to its use in treating stubborn acne, pigmentation, and dryness.

Folate, a B vitamin, and vitamin B_{12} are both essential for healthy, strong nails, and biotin, another B vitamin, is highly involved in the processes that create healthy, lustrous hair.

Great energy and vitality also contribute significantly to our sparkle, and the only way we are able to get the fuel out of our food is when we have optimal levels of B vitamins. Optimal B-vitamin levels allow us to make the most out of the food and nutrients we consume. With low vitamin-B levels, our food is unable to energize us effectively. B vitamins are essential to liver detoxification processes, critical for great skin, and are also vital to adrenal health, explored in detail in the Not-So-Beautiful Stress Hormones chapter.

Even though the B-group vitamins are found in many foods, they are water-soluble and delicate. They are easily destroyed, particularly by alcohol and cooking. Food processing can also reduce the amount of B-group vitamins in foods, making white flours, breads, and rice less nutritious than their whole grain counterparts.

The body has a limited capacity to store most of the B-group vitamins, except for B_{12} and folate, which are stored in the liver. A person who has a poor diet for a few months may end up with a B-group vitamin deficiency. Some low-carb diets also lead to a B-group vitamin deficiency. For this reason, it is important that adequate amounts of these vitamins be eaten regularly. Supplementation with a high-quality B-complex or multi-vitamin supplement has also been shown to be highly beneficial.

Good food sources of vitamin B_1 include seeds, particularly sesame seeds, legumes, nuts, savoury yeast, and pork. Whole grains are also a good source of vitamin B_1; however, many people today feel better without grains, or with only small amounts of grains, in their diet. If your digestion, for example, functions better without grains, try some gluten-free grains to see if they serve you better, and, if not, then go with what your body is guiding you to do. Just know that your dietary intake of vitamin B_1, or most likely all B vitamins, will be low and you will need to supplement.

Food sources of vitamin B_3 include meats, fish, chicken, eggs, whole grains, nuts, mushrooms, and almost all protein-containing foods.

Food sources of vitamin B_5 are widespread and found in a range of foods, but some good sources include eggs, meats, savoury yeast, and legumes.

Sources of biotin include eggs, chicken, savoury yeast, salmon, sardines, pork, avocado, cauliflower, mushrooms, raspberries, bananas, nuts (such as walnuts, almonds, and pecans), legumes, and whole grains. Food-processing methods destroy biotin so, like other B vitamins, unprocessed foods are a richer source of this nutrient.

Food sources of folate include green leafy vegetables, legumes, seeds, eggs, and citrus fruits. The only food sources of vitamin B_{12} are those of animal origin.

Vitamin B-deficiency signs are highly varied. Some of the most common and earlier signs include redness and irritation in the skin, particularly around the nose and mouth, cracks at the corners of the mouth, a dermatitis-type rash, particularly when under stress, and hypo- or hyper-pigmentation may occur with chronic low vitamin B-intake. With B_{12} and folate deficiencies, the nails take on a spoon shape. Instead of getting frustrated with your body if you don't like your nails or the cracks in the corners of your mouth that won't heal, use these signs as indicators that your body needs you to eat, drink, think, move, believe or perceive differently. When you listen and take action, not only will the bits that frustrate you clear up, but also many other bodily processes will be more efficient and healthier in the process.

Where do I start with this superstar nutrient? It is difficult to not play favourites with beautiful vitamin C! It does so many wonderful things for our health and beauty.

Vitamin C is highly effective at reducing free radical damage, such as that caused by overexposure to the sun or pollution. Free radicals consume collagen and elastin, promoting wrinkles and other signs of premature aging. Vitamin C is also involved in the production of collagen, not just the prevention of its breakdown, and, when combined with vitamin E, it is especially effective at protecting the skin from overexposure to the sun.

The health of your hair depends on vitamin C, as this vitamin supports the blood vessels that feed the hair follicles and is critical for circulation to the scalp.

Foods high in vitamin C include berries, capsicums (peppers), citrus fruits, kale, parsley, and broccoli. Signs of vitamin C-deficiency include premature aging, dull skin, dilated capillaries, and easy bruising. Hair that breaks easily is another sign that more vitamin C is needed in the diet.

You need vitamin C daily to help your body make collagen, the elastic tissue that is found in the skin, ligaments, tendons, cartilage, and blood vessels. It is also important for the growth and repair of your bones, teeth, and other tissues. Additionally, vitamin C is a powerful antioxidant that reduces damage and inflammation in the body, helping to protect you from degenerative diseases. I travel regularly for my work, and this is one nutrient I supplement daily.

Minerals and Trace Minerals

Minerals play vital roles in inner health and, therefore, outer beauty. Alkaline in nature, they help support a vast array of biochemical processes in the body. They also help balance your sex hormones, help your body relax, and promote happiness. Yet, today, I am deeply concerned that too many people don't get enough, let alone the optimal amounts of certain minerals. By definition, macro- minerals are those that the body requires 100 milligrams or more of per day, while trace or micro-minerals are those that the body requires in doses of less than 100 milligrams per day. Although we require smaller amounts of trace minerals, they are just as important to our health as macro-minerals. Let's explore those minerals that are intricately linked to your beauty.

CALCIUM

You are probably familiar with the role calcium plays in bone health, but many people are unaware of the extensive role it plays in countless other processes within the body. Our ability to absorb and distribute calcium throughout the body, for example, has an impact on the strength of our hair and nails.

Think this through. You consume a meal that contains some calcium. The calcium is extracted from the meal and is absorbed from your gut across and into your blood. That nutrient-rich blood then travels to the liver, and the liver assesses your body and decides where that calcium will best be used. (It is the liver that makes the decision where nutrients need to be dispersed to.) The liver will always send the calcium where it is needed most, and the place it is needed most is the task most necessary to keep you alive. For example, if you have been relying too much on processed food and caffeine, and churning out stress hormones, your blood needs the calcium to help maintain the pH. So rather than send the calcium to the "pretty areas", such as your nails or hair, your liver chooses elsewhere, knowing that your life is not dependent on your nails and hair being in their best shape. With this example, you can see how numerous processes critical to your beauty can be compromised when you are living on stress hormones as is so common today. For maximum calcium utilization, your diet needs to be nutrient-rich, high in plants, not reliant on processed foods, stress needs to be managed, and your digestive system needs to work well. Caffeine interferes with the absorption of calcium so, for some, nail health in particular will improve when caffeine consumption is decreased or at zero.

Food sources of calcium include green leafy vegetables, nuts, seeds (particularly sesame seeds), tahini, figs, and sardines. If you take a calcium supplement, the citrate form of calcium is well tolerated and absorbed, and it is good to take one that also contains magnesium, boron, and vitamin D, as all of these nutrients are essential for great bone health and nails.

MAGNESIUM

With the European Union recently authorizing a list of the associated health benefits of taking magnesium, it seems that this mineral itself has beautiful impacts both inside and out. Traditional Chinese medicine considers magnesium "the mineral of beauty", and it is the fourth most abundant mineral in the body, with around 50 per cent being found in our bones. This explains the connection between magnesium and bone density. What we don't read as much about are the other 300 or more biochemical reactions occurring in the body for which magnesium is an essential cofactor, meaning the reactions inside your body don't happen without it. Unfortunately, due to poor dietary habits, such as too much processed food and caffeine, pharmaceutical drug use, and nutrient-depleted soils, many people today are deficient in this essential mineral. Given the role magnesium plays in the proper functioning of nearly all of the systems of the body, this can have serious health and, therefore, beauty consequences. The health benefits of optimal magnesium intake include great energy (or certainly a reduction in fatigue), balanced electrolytes, which are essential for hydration and beautiful skin, boosted muscle and nervous system functioning, good protein synthesis, and maintenance of healthy teeth and strong bones. What a mineral!

The best food sources include leafy green vegetables, tahini, seeds, nuts, nut butter (such as almond butter), seaweed (such as kelp), and raw cacao. You can also supplement magnesium. The citrate form is well tolerated and easy for the body to absorb and utilize. You are also able to absorb magnesium through your skin. Taking a bath containing magnesium salts such as Epsom salts can be another way to enhance your magnesium levels. Because magnesium is a relaxant, if you have too much, your stools can become loose. If while supplementing you notice this, see this as a sign that you need less magnesium.

ZINC

What does this mineral *not* do? Zinc is another superstar among the nutrients, and it contributes to hundreds of processes inside your body, plenty of which are reflected on the outside.

Zinc is critical for wound healing. Whether that is a cut on your finger, the place where a surgical incision was made, or the aftermath of a pimple, zinc is necessary for the skin involved in these traumas to heal, and it helps prevent scar formation.

This mineral is an important component of healthy skin, especially for acne sufferers. Zinc acts by controlling the production of oil in the skin, and it also helps balance some of the hormones that can be involved in driving acne.

Zinc is required for proper immune system function, as well as for the maintenance of vision, taste, and smell. It is essential to the creation of over 300 enzymes necessary for you to have great digestion, the foundation of all health and beauty. Zinc even nourishes the scalp, helping to maintain the integrity and strength of hair, and low zinc levels have been linked with hair loss and a dry, flaky scalp.

As was indicated at the beginning of this chapter, if a nutrient is not in the soil, it cannot be in the food. Not even 100 years ago, zinc was abundant in many soils; therefore, fruit and vegetables were good sources of it. But because most soils in the world are now zinc-deficient, most foods do not contain zinc, unless they are grown in organic or biodynamically farmed soil. Many people today are deficient in this vital mineral that is responsible for the taste and texture of food, and may be contributing to why young children today tend to be fussier with food than in the past.

Foods that contain zinc include oysters from clean waters, eggs, red meat, pumpkin seeds, and sunflower seeds. Zinc can be supplemented and, if it is, because its absorption can be interfered with by many substances in food, including fibre, it is best taken before bed to maximize absorption.

Zinc deficiency signs can include white flecks in the nails, purple markings on the skin after breakouts or skin trauma, stretch marks that won't disappear, frequent colds and/or flu, hair loss, and a loss of appetite.

IRON

Iron is another mineral vital to your inner health and outer beauty, particularly your energy and hair, yet iron deficiency is the most common dietary deficiency in the world. It particularly affects children, menstruating women, and pregnant women. In New Zealand, it is estimated that up to 25 per cent of children under the age of three have some degree of iron deficiency, a deeply concerning statistic. According to the World Health Organization (WHO), a staggering 2 billion people in the world, in both developing and industrialized countries, are iron-deficient. Between 20 and 30 per cent of women of child-bearing age in Australia and New Zealand, research suggests, are iron-deficient.

Many people are confused about the difference between iron deficiency and another term you may have heard of, anaemia. Immature red blood cells require iron to be converted by the body into a form they can use in order to mature. When fully mature, they will become the oxygen carriers of the body, distributing oxygen from the lungs to all the other cells throughout the body. They have a big and important job to do!

Iron deficiency is the first step towards a decrease in the amount of oxygen-carrying, iron-rich haemoglobin within each red blood cell. As red blood cells are deprived of the quota of iron, they become contracted and smaller, known in medical terms as becoming microcytic. Anaemia develops when the immature red blood cells, deprived of their quota of iron, fail to survive their infancy. A formal diagnosis of anaemia is made when there is a consequent and significant decrease in the number of mature red blood cells.

Iron-deficiency anaemia is caused by inadequate dietary intake of iron, poor absorption of iron by the body, or loss of iron due to bleeding. Heavy menstrual blood loss is a common cause, as are increased demands for iron during pregnancy. In pregnant women, iron stores have to serve the increased blood volume of the mother, as well as the needs of the growing baby.

The condition can also be caused by blood loss from the digestive tract due to the long-term use of aspirin, or due to gastric ulcers, duodenal ulcers, bowel cancer, or untreated coeliac disease. I see more and more silent coeliac disease, where people are not presenting with the typical bowel symptoms. Sometimes iron deficiency, and often vitamin B_{12} deficiency, are the only signs of what is later diagnosed on biopsy as coeliac disease. Once gluten is removed from the diet, iron levels return to normal.

Fibre interferes with the absorption of dietary iron, so the fibre content of the diet must also be taken into account when determining the basis of the iron deficiency.

In the gut, calcium and iron compete for absorption, and calcium is a larger substance, so it always wins out. This is great news for your bones but not always so good for the oxygen-carrying capacity of your blood, low levels of which cause fatigue, which can take away from your shine. Consuming calcium-rich foods away from iron-rich foods can make a difference to iron absorption.

Iron is absolutely critical for great energy, sparkling eyes, and a vitality that lasts all day. The main symptoms of iron deficiency include exhaustion, shortness of breath, especially on an incline, muscle aches and cramps, rapid pulse and heart palpitations, increased anxiety, brain fog, poor memory and concentration, headaches, depressed mood, hair loss, and an increased frequency of infections. A simple blood test from your doctor will establish whether you are iron-deficient or not. Testing is important because some people have a tendency to store too much iron in the body and this needs to be avoided, or treated if it already exists.

Good food sources of iron include beef, lamb, eggs, mussels, sardines, lentils, and green leafy vegetables. Variety is key, as there is a small amount of iron in many foods. If you do not eat animal foods, do not assume you are iron-deficient. For some vegetarians, their body utilizes the iron from vegetables sources very efficiently. Vegetable sources of iron are better absorbed in the presence of vitamin C. It is best to have a test before you supplement. Many iron supplements are constipating, but most people find this does not happen with liquid iron supplements.

SILICA

Silica is a trace mineral that strengthens the body's connective tissues, which include muscles, tendons, hair, ligaments, nails, cartilage, and bone; and it is vital for healthy skin.

If your diet is lacking in silica, it can result in slackening of the skin and impaired wound healing. It can also mean weak nails and dull, brittle, and fine hair. Conversely, when your diet is sufficient in silica, you support great skin, thick, shiny hair, and strong nails, among other things.

Food sources include leeks, green beans, strawberries, cucumber, mango, celery, asparagus, rhubarb, apples, cabbage, carrots, cucumber, pumpkin, honey, fish, almonds, and oranges. Silica is also found in the horsetail herb and in bamboo leaf tea. Signs your body gives you that you may be deficient in silica include weak, brittle hair and nails and skin that are lacking in elasticity and firmness.

SELENIUM

There are more macro- and trace minerals than I am going into in this chapter, but there are some that are essential to focus on because of the role they play in beauty mechanisms. Selenium is one of those trace minerals, and I hope you will feel my love for this superstar bouncing off the page! Selenium's roles are vast and varied. It is an antioxidant mineral responsible for tissue elasticity, and it also acts to prevent free radical damage to cells. Research suggests that selenium may play an important role in preventing skin cancer, as it appears to protect the skin from damage from excessive ultraviolet light.

Selenium also benefits the skin as it assists the healing process. Selenium's antioxidant properties regenerate vitamins E and C, thereby decreasing the aging of skin. Other important benefits of selenium include boosting the immunological response against bacterial and viral infections, and against cancer cells, cold sores, and shingles. This important mineral also helps the body recycle and produce more glutathione (explored in moment). Selenium is also critical for fertility and optimal thyroid gland function, explored in more detail in the Beautiful Thyroid Hormones chapter.

The case of selenium highlights the critical nature of the quality of the soil. Most of the soil in Australia is deficient, as is the soil in New Zealand, the United Kingdom, and China, while soils in parts of the United States, Canada, and South America still contain some selenium. Remember, the food can't contain the mineral if it is not in the soil.

Current dietary sources of selenium include Brazil nuts, eggs, and brown rice. Small amounts are also found in some seafood and meat. Brazil nuts are perhaps the best source, although the amount of selenium in each nut varies. Research suggests that eating just three to six Brazil nuts per day provides adequate selenium intake for most people, and what a yummy way to get your selenium! The health benefits of selenium were another reason we based the Beetroot Chocolate Mudcake from the *Real Food Chef* cookbook on Brazil nuts. Now that's a delicious way to obtain your selenium!

Selenium deficiency can be hard to recognize through skin analysis; however, the skin will be prone to dryness and sensitivity, lacking radiance, with possible signs of premature aging. It more typically shows up as a compromised immune system and/or thyroid function, or through challenges with fertility.

Iodine's importance to overall health and well-being cannot be overstated. Iodine is critical for the formation of the thyroid hormones, which are so critical to our sparkle that I have devoted an entire chapter to your beautiful thyroid.

Iodine has many actions in the body. A shortage of iodine can cause changes to the thyroid gland that directly lead to poor metabolism and immunity. Iodine deficiency promotes free radical damage in the thyroid gland, which puts the gland itself at risk. Iodine blocks various compounds from binding to and accumulating in the thyroid gland, such as fluoride and goitrogens. Environmental pollution significantly aggravates an iodine lack and displaces iodine in the body.

There are high concentrations of iodine in the ovaries and breast tissue, where it acts as a buffer to the growth-stimulating effects of oestrogen, and promotes proper oestrogen metabolism. It assists the functioning of hormone receptors throughout the body, helping hormones communicate more effectively.

Iodine is essential for proper brain development and cognitive ability. There have been many studies showing the importance of iodine during gestation when cognitive potential is formed. The rapid rate of growth of the brain during the last trimester of pregnancy and the early postnatal stage makes it vulnerable to an inadequate diet. A deficiency of iodine during this critical period in brain development is associated with reduced intellectual ability. Iodine deficiency is the most common cause of preventable mental impairment worldwide.

Food sources of iodine include salt, although not all salt contains iodine. Himalayan pink salt and Celtic sea salt contain 84 different minerals, and in most brands one of these is iodine. It is best to check the label to be sure. Seaweeds, such as kelp and nori, are another good source of iodine. You can add seaweeds, such as kombu, to soups, stews, and casseroles to impart a lovely salty flavour as well as some iodine, and remove the stick of seaweed before serving. Iodine can also be supplemented in the diet.

Iodine deficiency can lead to dull and brittle hair, balding, lack of skin tone and/or very dry skin, low energy levels, difficulty dealing with environmental temperature change so much so that you feel "cold in your bones" and find it difficult to warm up, poor concentration, constipation, depressed mood, puffy eyes, and extreme fatigue.

Fats

I have already waxed lyrical about the immense benefits of certain fats in the diet, especially with regards to the appearance of your skin, but there are some fats that deserve special mention in this Beautiful Nutrients chapter. They are what are called the essential fatty acids (EFAs), of which there are omega-3 and omega-6 types. They are literally essential, meaning they have to be consumed daily for us to be well, on the inside and outside, as we cannot create them from other fats we eat or generate. The others fats that deserve special mention when it comes to inner health and outer beauty are the medium-chain triglycerides, in particular lauric acid.

ESSENTIAL FATTY ACIDS: OMEGA-3 AND OMEGA-6

The omega-3 fats that must be consumed daily are eicosapentaenoic acid (EPA) and docosahexaenoic acid (DHA), which the body can convert from another essential fatty acid called alpha-linolenic acid (ALA), which also must be consumed. However, the conversion of ALA into the critical EPA and DHA fats is inefficient in some people. Hence, it is wise to include adequate amounts of all of these fats in your diet. The health benefits of EPA and DHA are well documented; they are powerful anti-inflammatories, making them highly beneficial to the skin. They take up residence in the membrane (outside layer) of the cell and are able to exert their anti-inflammatory effects and keep the cells flexible. Due to their physical structure (which contains double bonds), they themselves oxidize easily and are best consumed with an antioxidant-rich diet.

The omega-6 essential fatty acid is called linoleic acid (LA), which the body elongates (converts) into the vital gamma linolenic acid (GLA). GLA can also be consumed, a necessary dietary action if people are inefficient at converting LA into GLA. This is usually true for people with eczema; their skin does better having the GLA supplied directly.

Dry, inflamed skin, or skin that suffers from the frequent appearance of whiteheads or blackheads, can benefit from supplementing with EFAs. They play a major role in skin repair, moisture content, and overall flexibility, but, as you now understand, because the body cannot produce its own EFAs, they must be obtained through the diet. The typical Western diet is overabundant in omega-6 fatty acids — which are found in many processed foods, baked goods, and grains — and lacking in omega-3s. DHA is found in cold-water fish, such as salmon and mackerel, while the other omega-3 fat, EPA, is found in flaxseeds, chia seeds, and walnuts. A good choice in the omega-6 EFA category is evening primrose oil, which contains GLA and has been shown to help people with eczema take up fat into their skin, allowing it to soften and be moisturized.

Balancing the intake of omega-6 fats with omega-3s can result in smoother, younger-looking skin. Countless people have commented to me that when they focus on increasing the EFA content of their diet through food and/or supplementation, after only a few weeks they can feel and notice a difference in the softness of their skin.

As I mentioned, you can supplement your diet with EFAs. I have seen great results for health and skin when a food-based, liquid fatty acid that contains a variety of plant-based oils is used in addition to a real food diet, high in antioxidants.

Some EFA deficiency signs include dandruff, dull skin, dry skin, cracked heels (on the feet), skin sensitivity, keratosis pilaris, which are tiny dots often described as a "chicken skin" appearance on the backs of the arms and legs (which can also be caused by too much fruit in the diet).

MEDIUM-CHAIN TRIGLYCERIDES

All fats and oils are composed of fat molecules called fatty acids, and there are two methods of classifying fatty acids. The one you are most probably most familiar with is based on saturation. There are saturated fatty acids, monounsaturated fatty acids, and polyunsaturated fatty acids. The second method of classification is based on molecular size or length of the carbon chain in the fatty acid. There are short-chain fatty acids (SCFA), medium-chain fatty acids (MCFA), and long-chain fatty acids (LCFA). Another term you will often see in reference to fatty acids is triglyceride. Three fatty acids joined together make a triglyceride, so you may have short-chain triglycerides (SCT), medium-chain triglycerides (MCT), or long-chain triglycerides (LCT).

The vast majority of the fats and oils you eat — whether they are saturated or unsaturated, or come from an animal or a plant — are composed of long-chain triglycerides. Probably 98–100 per cent of all the fats most people eat consist of LCT. However, some food, such as coconut, is rather unique as it is composed predominately of MCT. Organic butter also contains some MCTs.

MCTs are broken down almost immediately by enzymes in the saliva and gastric juices so that pancreatic fat-digesting enzymes are not even essential for their digestion, which is great for people who experience challenges with their digestive system. In the digestive system, MCTs are broken down into individual fatty acids (MCFA). Unlike other fatty acids, MCFAs are absorbed directly from the intestines into the portal vein (a vein that goes straight to the liver) and sent straight to the liver where they are, for the most part, burned as fuel.

Other fats require pancreatic enzymes to break them into smaller units. They are then absorbed into the intestinal wall and packaged into bundles of fat (lipid) and protein called lipoproteins. These lipoproteins are carried by the lymphatic system, bypassing the liver, and then dumped into the bloodstream, where they are circulated throughout the body. As they circulate in the blood, their fatty components are distributed to all the tissues of the body. The lipoproteins get smaller and smaller, until there is little left of them. At this time, they are picked up by the liver, broken apart, and used to produce energy or, if needed, repackaged into other lipoproteins and sent back into the bloodstream to be distributed throughout the body. Cholesterol, saturated fat, monounsaturated fat, and polyunsaturated fat are all packaged together into lipoproteins and carried throughout the body in this way. In contrast, medium-chain fatty acids are not packaged into lipoproteins but go to the liver where they are converted into energy. Since medium-chain fatty acids tend to primarily produce energy, they are less likely to be stored to any significant degree as body fat.

One MCFA deserves special mention and that is lauric acid. As mentioned in the Beautiful Foods chapter, this incredible fat has powerful antibacterial and antifungal properties, with research showing it can be 15 times more powerful than benzoyl peroxide, the active ingredient in many acne medications and face washes, when it comes to killing the bacteria involved in acne. Both coconut and butter contain lauric acid. As an aside, butter from pasture-fed cows also contains conjugated linoleic acid (CLA), a relative of LA, which research has shown to have both anti-cancer properties as well as anti-inflammatory actions.

Additional Antioxidants

GLUTATHIONE

Glutathione has been regarded as the superhero of antioxidants, yet many people have never heard of it. Glutathione is a very simple molecule that is produced naturally all the time in your body. It is a combination of three building blocks of protein, or more precisely the amino acids cysteine, glycine, and glutamine. Normally, glutathione is recycled in the body, except when the toxic load becomes too great, which unfortunately is occurring more frequently for people these days, due to poor dietary and lifestyle choices as well as environmental exposure to pollutants. Glutathione is also reduced in many chronic diseases including diabetes.

It is so important because its main role is to recycle antioxidants. It is considered a master antioxidant as it works to support the other antioxidants. Free radicals can be generated from everyday metabolic processes, exposure to toxins and household chemicals, and they can inflict damage upon other compounds by stealing electrons from them, which initiates bouts of inflammation. To defend and protect the tissues of the body, the free radicals get passed around antioxidants, often from vitamin C to vitamin E, to lipoic acid and then finally to glutathione which cools off the free radicals, and recycles other antioxidants. After this happens, the body can reduce or regenerate another protective glutathione molecule. Isn't that incredible?

However, problems occur when we are overwhelmed with too much oxidative stress, including toxins. Glutathione can become depleted and we can no longer protect ourselves against free radicals and infections; our ability to eliminate toxins is impaired. Glutathione is the most critical and integral part of our detoxification systems. All the toxins stick onto glutathione, which then carries them into the bile, and eventually they are excreted from the body in stools. Glutathione has also been researched due to its ability to help us reach peak mental and physical function. Research suggests that raised glutathione levels decrease muscle damage, reduce recovery time, increase strength and endurance, and shift metabolism from fat production to muscle development. When glutathione production is impaired, you are lacking a powerful and natural ability to recover.

Here are some ways to stimulate glutathione production:

- **Consume sulphur-rich foods:** The main ones in the diet are garlic, onions, and the cruciferous vegetables, including broccoli, kale, cabbage, cauliflower, and watercress.

- **Exercise moderately:** This stimulates glutathione, which then helps boost your immune system, improves detoxification, and enhances your body's own antioxidant defences. Start slow and build up to 30 minutes a day. Strength training for 20 minutes three times a week is also helpful. In the Beautiful Posture and Movement chapter, I will offer guidance on choosing the right movement activities for your body.

- **Supplement with alpha-lipoic acid:** The body usually makes it, but, given all the stresses we are under, we often become depleted. Supplementing with alpha-lipoic acid can help (see below).

- **Methylating nutrients (vitamins B_6 and B_{12}):** These nutrients are perhaps the most critical to glutathione production. Methylation and the production and recycling of glutathione are two of the most important biochemical functions in your body.

- **Consume optimal amounts of selenium:** This important mineral helps the body recycle and produce more glutathione.

- **Consume optimal amounts of vitamins C and E:** These vitamins work together to recycle glutathione. Include vitamin C-rich fruits and vegetables in your diet for your vitamin C, and eat almonds to help increase your vitamin E.

- **Consume milk thistle (silymarin):** This herb has long been used by medical herbalists to support liver function; it also helps boost glutathione levels.

ALPHA-LIPOIC ACID

Alpha-lipoic acid has a wide range of benefits, the most important being its role as an antioxidant. In 1988, it was discovered that alpha-lipoic acid has powerful antioxidant abilities, equal to that of coenzyme Q_{10}, vitamin C, and vitamin E.

Unlike other antioxidants, alpha-lipoic acid has the unique ability to neutralize free radicals within aqueous (water-based) and lipid (fatty) regions of cells, as well as in intracellular and extracellular environments. This ability allows alpha-lipoic acid to be easily transported across cellular membranes to neutralize free radicals. Vitamin C is only able to protect the watery portions of cells from free radical attack, and vitamin E is only able to protect the fatty membranes. But alpha-lipoic acid has the ability to neutralize free radicals that occur in both the watery and fatty regions of the cell. Alpha-lipoic acid is capable of neutralizing a wide variety of free radicals, such as singlet oxygen, superoxides, peroxyl and hydroxyl radicals, hypochlorite, and peroxynitrite — all names you don't need to worry about remembering! Just know that other antioxidants, like vitamin

C, vitamin E, or glutathione, can only neutralize one kind of free radical. Researchers often refer to alpha-lipoic acid as the universal antioxidant because it can neutralize such a wide variety of free radicals.

Not only is alpha-lipoic acid able to neutralize free radicals, it is also able to recycle or regenerate several other important antioxidants, including vitamin C and glutathione. When an antioxidant scavenges a free radical, it becomes oxidized in the process and is not able to scavenge additional free radicals until it has been reduced (saved). The reduced form of alpha-lipoic acid, called dihydro-lipoic acid, is able to reduce the oxidized antioxidants, enabling them to be useful again. I love how clever alpha-lipoic acid is.

Because of its antioxidant activity, alpha-lipoic acid is wonderful for your skin and for slowing the aging process. Your body is able to synthesize some alpha-lipoic acid.

Alpha-lipoic acid is found in abundance in animal tissues with high metabolic activity, such as kidney, heart, and liver, and, to a lesser extent, in fruits and vegetables. Non-animal sources are spinach, broccoli, tomatoes, peas, and Brussels sprouts. All alpha-lipoic acid supplied by the diet is transported in the bloodstream to tissues and incorporated into cells. It is then transferred into the mitochondria, which are the energy powerhouses of the cell. Studies in mammals have shown the alpha-lipoic acid supplied by the diet does not supply enough for purposes such as incorporation into enzyme complexes. Hence, these sources of alpha-lipoic acid are thought to provide very little free alpha-lipoic acid into circulation. It is only through supplementation that alpha-lipoic acid has been shown to reach potentially therapeutic levels.

COENZYME Q_{10}

Coenzyme Q_{10} (CoQ_{10}), another powerful antioxidant, is a substance that is found naturally in almost every cell in the body; it helps convert food into energy. As you now know, antioxidants are critical to our health, longevity, and beauty, as they couple with free radicals, which have the ability, if left unattached, to damage cell membranes, tamper with DNA, and even cause cell death. As you also know, free radicals contribute to the aging process, as well as to a number of health problems, including heart disease and cancer. Antioxidants, such as CoQ_{10}, can neutralize free radicals and may reduce or even help prevent some of the damage they cause. Research has shown that CoQ_{10} may help with heart-related conditions, because it can improve energy production in cells, prevent blood-clot formation, and act as an antioxidant. Its anti-aging effects have also been noted on skin. Here are some ways CoQ_{10} has been shown to impact positively on skin.

Young skin has ample amounts of CoQ_{10}, and therefore lots of energy, and energy is needed to repair damage and make sure the skin cells are healthy. CoQ_{10} has been shown to protect against photo-aging, premature aging due to overexposing the skin to the sun. CoQ_{10} may rejuvenate skin by stimulating skin cell activity. Active skin cells get rid of toxins easily and can make better use of nutrients. When your skin ages, all of these processes slow down, causing dull, sallow, and wrinkled skin. CoQ_{10} counteracts this by stimulating collagen production. As a reminder, collagen is the protein that tends to decrease as we age, leading to wrinkles and leathery skin. And as CoQ_{10} is a potent antioxidant, it, importantly for your beauty, acts against oxidative damage. This damage is done by, for example, UV rays of the sun, pollutants, and stress. Damage all leads to one thing: premature aging that shows up on the skin. When metals oxidise, we call it rust. When humans oxidise, we call it aging! Sometimes too much oxidation can lead to disease, so we need something to help prevent us from "rusting". And antioxidants do just that.

Food sources include fish and brown rice. Organ meats, such as liver, heart and kidney, also contain CoQ10, and it is readily available as a supplement.

Elements Unique to Plants

Specific plant foods contain powerful substances that can be very healing to your skin. Like antioxidants, these chemicals boost the immune system and help slow the aging process from the inside out. In time, science will discover more and more about the magic of Mother Nature and thousands more of these unique compounds will be found. Here are two with particularly powerful properties.

FLAVONOIDS

Flavonoids are found in abundance in a wide range of fruits and vegetables, including apples, cranberries, tomatoes, celery, kale, parsley, as well as in green and black tea. They help cool inflammation, slow and even cease oxidation, and thereby help protect your skin from aging and wrinkling. Flavonoids have also been shown to support the immune system, suppress the growth of tumours, and prevent blood clots — even more reasons to amp up the plant content of your diet.

INDOLES

These amazing phytochemical substances are found in cruciferous vegetables such as broccoli, cauliflower, kale, Brussels sprouts, and cabbage. They behave like antioxidants, reduce inflammation, and have been shown to support healthy oestrogen metabolism (something you will see in the Beautiful Sex Hormones chapter), which is crucial for health and beauty, and to reduce the risk of developing reproductive cancers.

Nutrients: A Summary

You can see from the explanations above that all nutrients are essential to your inner health and outer beauty, and even if only one is deficient in the diet, there are both visible and "silent" consequences. I cannot encourage you enough to obtain as many nutrients as possible from your food, and when your diet is mostly real food and high in plants you have the opportunity to maximize every mouthful. Make this what you do. However, the nutrient density of the food you eat is dependent on the quality of the soil in which it is grown, and as a consumer you aren't always, if ever, aware of where your food has come from, let alone the quality of soil that contributed to its growth. Supplements do not make up for a poor-quality diet, as there are compounds present in whole foods that are unique in their ability to support your health. Yet the world we live in is different to the one our grandparents inhabited. More is demanded of many people's biochemistry, including from constantly elevated stress hormones due to the pace of life as well as from technology. Plus we are exposed to more pollutants — from sources such as the number of cars on the road to the pesticides on conventionally grown foods that didn't even exist 100 years ago — requiring more detoxification than ever before. Nutritional supplements can therefore play a highly beneficial role in supporting optimal inner health and outer shine.

The parts of your body that frustrate or sadden you are simply messengers asking you to eat, drink, move, think, believe or perceive in a new way. See them as the gift that they are.

Dr Libby

Chapter 3

Beautiful Hydration:

the wonder of water

Water is the basis of all life, and that includes your body. The muscles that move your body are 75 per cent water. Your blood, responsible for transporting nutrients throughout your body, is 82 per cent water. Your lungs, that take oxygen from the air, are 90 per cent water, while your brain is 76 per cent water. Even your bones are 25 per cent water!

Most people are aware of the critical importance of great hydration for their health, and of course for their skin in particular. But few people truly understand what beautiful hydration is and how to ensure it. Scientists believe that when we are born we are about 75 per cent water, but by the time we are 30 most adults' total body water content has dropped to around 57–60 per cent. I will use 70 per cent as an average to make this discussion simple. Think about this concept: 70 per cent of your physical body is water. Wow. No wonder the impact of dehydration is significant on our inner health and outer sparkle.

Our health is truly dependent on the quality and quantity of the water we drink. Unintentional chronic dehydration can contribute to pain and inflammation in the body, and it can even be involved in the development of many degenerative diseases. Helping your body prevent such ills by ensuring great-quality water intake on a regular basis is a crucial step with any health and/or beauty focus.

Here is an article I wrote for a magazine in New Zealand, which is useful to include here.

The Wonder of Water: The Key to Happy, Healthy Cells

When it comes to water, most people believe they need to drink more than they currently do, and, without a conscious effort, this never seems to happen. The wonders of water are well documented, ranging from fostering glowing, clear skin and eyes to the prevention of kidney stones. Yet, as with most nutritional information, there is conflicting information out there, which makes it difficult for individuals to truly know how much is enough.

The Science

Without water, a human will usually only live for a mere three days. So essential is this liquid to our survival that we need it more than food. Science currently tells us that we need 33 millilitres (mL) of water for each kilogram (kg) of our body weight. A

70kg person, therefore, requires 2310mL (2.31 litres) a day. We do, however, tend to forget that many plant foods have a high water content, and this contributes to our overall daily water consumption. Herbal teas and soups also add up. Foods and drinks containing caffeine and alcohol, however, draw water out of our body, so the larger their presence in our diet, the greater our fluid requirements.

Fruits and vegetables are almost always over 70 per cent water, so the more of these we eat, the less we need to consume as fluid. Naturally, perspiration and increased breathing rates generated by exercise increase our need for water, but the specific amounts necessary are difficult to determine and will be highly individual. Trust your thirst when it comes to this. Thirst is Nature's way of letting you know you need to drink!

Thirst and Hydration

Some people rarely feel thirsty, while for others their thirst never seems quenched. Some people resist increasing their fluid intake as they tire of frequently running to the loo. Yet, for others, increasing their fluid intake makes them feel swollen and uncomfortable. With all of these different scenarios, it is not surprising that there is so much conflicting information out there. So what's behind these differences and what can you do about it?

Just because you drink water, or even enough water for adequate hydration, does not necessarily mean that the cells of your body are hydrated. Ideally, every cell of your body looks like a grape; this is the case when your cells are hydrated. A dehydrated state means your cells appear more like sultanas, and this can be the result of inadequate water intake, a lack of minerals, or poor adrenal gland function, often due to chronic stress, physical and/or emotional trauma, or excess caffeine or alcohol.

To absorb the water you drink into your cells, you need calcium, magnesium, sodium, potassium, and chloride. Some of these minerals make their home inside the cell, while others reside outside the cell wall. These minerals all talk to each other, and if one has an excessively high level or, alternatively, if one of those minerals is lacking, it can be difficult for water to enter the cell. Physically, when water stays outside the cell, it manifests as a feeling of fluid retention, which, for some people, is so noticeable that clothing will cut into them as the day progresses. You can change this by improving the mineral balance of your diet and taking care of your liver.

One of the best ways to improve your mineral intake and balance is to base your diet on what I have come to call low Human Intervention (HI) food. Most plant foods get their minerals from the soil in which they are grown, so foods that come from organic, biodynamic, or permacultured soils tend to be superior in their mineral profile. Green leafy vegies have a broad mineral profile that includes calcium, magnesium, and potassium. Nuts and seeds also pack a powerful mineral punch and make a great snack or addition to any meal.

Minerals

People with low blood pressure often feel better with a slightly reduced fluid intake, as excess water dilutes their blood levels of minerals. Increasing your intake of all of the minerals above can, however, *make a significant difference in that low blood pressure feeling.*

Your body uses minerals to, among other things, create electrolytes. Often described as the sparks of life, electrolytes carry electrical currents through the body, sending instructions to cells in all body systems. Electrolytes are also necessary for enzyme production. Enzymes are responsible the biochemical processes that drive the function of the body, as well as for digesting food, absorbing nutrients, and they impact both muscle function and hormone production as well. Poor mineral intake and/or balance as well as dehydration, therefore, affect all body systems and functions.

Amp Up Your Mineral Intake

A healthy and balanced way to increase the amount of minerals in your diet is to amp up the amount of plant foods you currently consume, the green-coloured ones in particular. Add them wherever you can, and do your best to base your evening meal on greens, rather than them being a token effort on the side of the plate. You can also include Celtic sea salt or Himalayan pink salt. They typically contain 84 minerals that can help your body better absorb water into the cells. Adding good-quality salt to your food can be of particular importance if you eat limited or no processed foods, particularly if you suffer with digestive system problems.

Juicing or blending fruits and vegetables is also a great way to increase the fluid and mineral content of your diet and ensure that water is absorbed into your cells. If fluid retention is an ongoing challenge for you, try juicing celery, cucumber, mint, and a small amount of pineapple daily for a week. Supplementing with a "green drink" supplement such as barley grass can also be beneficial.

Another way to gently increase the mineral content of your diet is to choose water with a pH greater than eight. The pH level of water is displayed on the side of the bottle. The higher the pH, the higher the mineral content. New Zealand is incredibly fortunate with the wonderful range of alkaline water on offer that is sourced here, so if you buy water, choose those with a higher pH. For optimal digestion, remember to drink water between meals, rather than with meals, as water can dilute the power of your stomach acid necessary for the optimal digestion of your food.

Set up rituals in your day to flag your memory that it is time to drink. Start your day with a glass of warm water with lemon juice, for example. Make drinking enough natural water a habit in your life. It won't take long for you to feel the benefits. Water is a simple and wonderful investment in your long-term health.

~~~~~~~~~~~~~~~~~~~~~~~~

SUPPORT YOUR KIDNEYS, SUPPORT YOUR SKIN

The primary job of the kidneys is to remove the waste products of protein metabolism from the blood. These include nitrogen, uric acid (urea), and ammonia. The kidneys also remove many other substances from the blood that could become problematic if left to accumulate, including excess hormones, food additives, vitamins, minerals, and drugs. They also regulate the electrolyte balance of the body, which involves the minerals needed for healthy nerve function. These include calcium, magnesium, phosphate, sodium, potassium, and chloride. The kidneys also help regulate healthy blood pressure.

As you now understand, the kidneys regulate the amount of water in the body, and your urine is your blood having been filtered by the kidneys. Water plays an enormous role in keeping the moisture content of our skin at a lovely high level. Consuming adequate water also helps to promote healthy elimination, and it reduces the likelihood of constipation, as one of the primary functions of the large intestine is to absorb water from digested food. When water consumption is low, stools tend to become dry, hard, and more difficult to pass, and the longer this waste remains inside the body, the more waste will be reabsorbed back into the bloodstream, through which it soon finds its way to the skin. The importance of great elimination and detoxification are discussed in detail in later chapters.

It is obvious then, that if we are to have beautiful, well-hydrated skin, we must take good care of our kidneys. Here's how to support their optimal function:

✓ Drink adequate amounts of pure water each day. Keep a large glass at your desk to ensure you stay hydrated over the day. Let your body guide you on how much water it needs by noticing your response to the water you drink. As you drink, observe if your thirst becomes awakened and your body actually seems to draw in the water. This is your body letting you know that it needs more water. Sometimes I start drinking and want another glass immediately. At other times, I am satisfied with one glass or a few sips. Give your body all the water it needs throughout the day to ensure that the elimination of waste via the urine is well supported. It is also important to minimize, or omit, your consumption of soft drinks and alcohol. If you have any type of skin condition, this is even more critical, and is particularly important for children and teenagers.

✓ Sleep well! You will notice that when you are exhausted, not only does everything feel more difficult, but your skin is also less radiant and more prone to breakouts, blemishes, and rashes. Rest and sleep strengthen the kidneys. Seven to nine hours of restorative sleep per night allows the kidneys to adequately cleanse the blood, eliminating waste products in the morning urine that would otherwise be shunted to the skin for excretion. Do all you can to establish a consistent rhythm between your sleeping and waking hours, particularly if you'd like more vitality. Consider taking a short nap on the weekends, especially when you are going through times of stress, which for many people these days is every week!

✓ Take part in regular restorative movement such as t'ai chi, qigong, yoga, and/or restorative yoga. These practices not only have specific poses or movements to support healthy kidney function, but the diaphragmatic breathing they foster is a powerful tool to decrease stress hormone production, explained in detail later in this book.

Integrity reveals beauty.

Thomas Leonard

Chapter 4
Beautiful Hormones:
their role in and impact on your shine

When it comes to radiant beauty, the biochemistry of the endocrine system is a key influencer on how you look, feel, and experience life. Here is a little bit of science made simple to help you on your way through this chapter. This knowledge, combined with the juicy bits that come later, will lead you to the aha moments that have the potential to transform your life, and deeply enhance your shine.

THE ENDOCRINE GLANDS: THE HORMONE SECRETORS

The endocrine system is made up of numerous glands that secrete hormones, including the pituitary, thyroid, parathyroids, and adrenals, as well as those involved in reproduction — the ovaries in women and the testes in men, although these are technically not endocrine glands exclusively. For the purpose of explaining the role of the endocrine system in beauty, though, the ovaries are included here, since they play a vital role in how we feel and function on a daily basis.

Around the age of 12, as they enter puberty, boys and girls start to develop striking differences in physical appearance and behaviour. Perhaps no other period in life so clearly demonstrates the impact of both the nervous system and the endocrine system in directing development and regulating body functions. Changes in the brain and pituitary gland markedly increase the synthesis of new messenger molecules, the sex hormones, from the gonads. In girls, fatty tissue starts to accumulate in the breasts and on the hips. At the same time or a little later, in boys protein synthesis increases, muscle mass builds, and the longer, larger vocal cords start producing a lower-pitched voice. These changes provide just a few examples of the powerful influence of the secretions from endocrine glands.

COORDINATION OF THE NERVOUS SYSTEM AND THE ENDOCRINE SYSTEM

The nervous system and the endocrine system work together to coordinate the functions of all of the body's systems. The nervous system controls homeostasis — the point where all things are in balance — through nerve impulses, while the endocrine system releases its messenger molecules — called hormones — into the bloodstream. The circulating blood then delivers hormones to virtually all cells throughout the body. The nervous and endocrine systems are coordinated as an interlocking super-system, referred to as the neuroendocrine system. Certain parts of the nervous system stimulate or inhibit the release of hormones from the glands of the endocrine system. Hormones may then, in turn, promote or inhibit the generation of nerve impulses. Also, several molecules act as hormones in some locations and as neurotransmitters in others.

The nervous system causes muscles to contract and glands to secrete more or less of their products. The endocrine system alters metabolic activities, regulates growth and development, and guides reproductive processes. It therefore not only helps regulate the activity of things like smooth and cardiac muscle and some glands, it significantly affects virtually all other tissues in the body as well.

Nerve impulses tend to produce their effects within milliseconds. While some hormones can act within seconds, others can take up to several hours or more to bring about their responses. Also, the effects of stimulating the nervous system are generally brief compared with those of the endocrine system.

So with that out of the way, let's get into the details of how the biochemistry of your endocrine system affects you; how you feel, look, and function every day.

Housed inside a part of your brain, the pituitary gland is the master gland, or switch, of the endocrine system. Technically, the hypothalamus, an organ with some endocrine tissue within it, influences the function of the pituitary; however, for ease of explanation and to keep the *Beauty from the Inside Out* message concise, the hypothalamus won't be explored in detail. It is briefly discussed in the Beautiful Thyroid and Beautiful Pituitary chapters within this Beautiful Hormones section.

The pituitary gland sends the signals out to your other endocrine system glands, alerting them to the hormones they need to make. Likewise, the thyroid talks to the ovaries. The adrenals and the ovaries also have a relationship, and on and on the chatter inside you goes. That's what hormones do: they talk, they send messages, and each of those messages communicates information to the different cells, tissues, and organs inside your body. Nothing, and I mean nothing, works alone. Everything is influenced by something else.

So the importance of the coming sections — about the adrenal glands and the stress hormones they make, the ovaries and the sex hormones they produce, the thyroid gland and the temperature-controlling, metabolism-influencing hormones it makes, as well as the master of them all, the pituitary — is enormous. They will open your mind and your heart to a whole new way to view your health, body, and beauty, as well as provide you with insights and support to make the changes you feel inspired to make. Hormones, here we come!

People often say that beauty is in the eye of the beholder, and I say that the most liberating thing about beauty is realizing that you are the beholder.

Salma Hayek

Chapter 4
Part 1

Not-So-Beautiful Stress Hormones:

the critical role of calm in your beauty

When it comes to substances inside your body that can take away your shine, stress hormones, when produced consistently and over extended periods, can have a pronounced and visible impact. Stress hormones themselves can interfere with your sparkle, and they have a significant impact on whether your sex hormones are balanced or not, which, as you will see from the next section, is critical to everything from your skin to your shine, your menstruation to your mood.

When I first started to work with people on their health, consultations were comparatively calm. Fifteen years ago, women would arrive mostly on time, relatively unhurried, and if they had a cell phone they turned it off. Now, often they rush in, their energy exuding impatience and urgency until at least 15 minutes into the consultation, their cell phones ring and ping with calls and emails, and, if I could make a sound that described them, it would be a high-pitched whizzing whir. Yes, I am generalizing, and of course some women put their phones on silent for our session. However, I am describing a general trend to make a point. Women are stretched and stressed and time-poor like never before. Of course we can argue that there has always been stress, but it has never before come in the constant, urgent avalanche that has become the norm for so many women in the Western world.

THE THREE PARTS OF THE BRAIN

Central to our response to stress is what is known as the fight-or-flight response: when faced with a perceived threat to our safety, we either stand our ground and meet the threat head-on, or we flee to safety. Our body's — and in particular our hormones' — response to perceived stress is influenced by the three integrated parts of the human brain. So we will briefly look at these before moving on to "stress in action".

The first part is the brain stem, or reptile brain. This is the *survival brain*. It controls the functions responsible for our survival, as an individual and as a species — such things as hunger, thirst, heart-beat, breathing, digestion, immunity, and sex drive. It is the basic, primal part of us that is in all animals; give me food, give me shelter, let me reproduce! This part of the brain also *initiates* the fight-or-flight stress response.

Our second part is the limbic system, or mammal brain. All mammals have it, and it is composed of the amygdala, hippocampus, and thalamus. This is our *emotional brain*. It controls all of the functions related to emotional aspects of survival, such as memory, behaviour, pleasure and pain responses, and our experience of all emotions. It *maintains* the fight-or-flight stress response.

The third part is the cerebral cortex, or human brain. Humans and some other mammals, such as apes, dolphins, and whales, have this brain, and it is our *thinking brain*. It controls such things as decision-making, attention, awareness, language, judgment, reading, and writing. It is the centre of higher thought and it is *impaired* by the fight-or-flight stress response.

These comprise the mental processes that feed into our physiological response to life. Now we will explore these physiological mechanisms in more detail, but later in the chapter we will return to the mental and physical partnership when we look at coping mechanisms.

THE ADRENAL GLANDS

Let's look at what we ask of our body from an adrenal and stress hormone perspective when we live a high-stress, high-paced lifestyle. For those of you who have read *Accidentally Overweight* and *Rushing Woman's Syndrome*, some of this information was covered there, but this section has been expanded and is essential reading at this stage in the *Beauty from the Inside Out* journey. My goal is to help you appreciate the powerful role that your adrenal glands play in your health, body shape and size, your vitality, your skin, hair, and nails, as well as how they contribute to your sense of coping and calm.

Your adrenal glands are two very precious, walnut-sized glands that sit just on top of your kidneys. They may be small, but the power they pack when they are working optimally is an energetic, vitality-inducing, health gift to us all. The adrenal glands produce many hormones, two of which are your stress hormones, namely adrenalin (epinephrine) and cortisol.

ADRENALIN, SUGAR CRAVINGS AND YOUR SHINE

Adrenalin is your short-term, acute stress hormone. It is the one that is produced when you get a fright. If someone suddenly runs into the room and startles you, the feeling that follows is caused by adrenalin. Adrenalin is designed to get you out of danger — and get you out of danger fast. Historically, humans made adrenalin when their lives were threatened. The response, fuelled by adrenalin, was typically physical. If a tiger suddenly jumped out of the jungle, or perhaps a member of another tribe started chasing you with a spear, the body made adrenalin, promoting the fight-or-flight response. When activated, the typically excellent blood supply to your digestive system is diverted away from your digestive system to your periphery, to your arms and your legs. This is necessary because you need a powerful blood supply to your arms and legs to get you out of danger. You also need fuel to help you escape, and the most readily available, fastest-burning fuel inside the body is glucose, often referred to as sugar, a carbohydrate. Your liver and muscles store glucose in the form of glycogen, and adrenalin communicates to your liver and muscles when energy is required. They then convert glycogen back into glucose and dump this glucose into your blood. Your blood sugar subsequently shoots up, ready to fuel your self-defence or your escape. And you feel amped up.

This cascade of events — and the biochemical changes that result — allows you to escape from danger in a very active way. Regardless of the outcome, regardless of whether you win that challenge or not (you escape, die, or win the fight), this stress, the threat to your life, and the need for adrenalin is over quickly. The trouble is that for many of us in the modern world, it is more often psychological stress that drives us to make adrenalin, and for many women today that stress is never switched off. Although our life may not literally be threatened, this hormone still communicates to every cell of our body that our life is indeed at risk. Adrenalin makes your heart race, your thoughts race, and gives you a jittery feeling that can make it difficult to feel calm and centred, despite your best efforts.

Psychological stress can come in many forms. It may be that you return from a week away from work to find 700 new emails in your in-box, and you wonder when on Earth you are going to find the time to deal with those. It may be that your landline rings and, while you take that call, your mobile rings, and you feel that you can barely finish one conversation before demands come in to start another one. If you are sitting in front of your computer while all of this is going on, and a few emails arrive in your in-box while you juggle the incoming demands and noise, adrenalin tends to climb higher. Or perhaps you set your alarm for the morning, you press the snooze button … you keep pressing snooze … and suddenly you sit bolt upright in bed and realize you are running late. Maybe you still have clothes to iron, lunches to prepare, little people to deliver to school, and, because you are leaving later than usual, you get stuck in traffic. Meanwhile, your mobile phone starts ringing with people at the office wondering where you are as you are supposed to be in a meeting, but you are stuck in the middle of rush-hour traffic, and your brain has gone into overdrive with the enormity of your morning. And you have only been up for an hour!

When you finally burst through the doors at work, all you can think about is how much you want a coffee. So all morning you have been making adrenalin, and now you are going to make even more adrenalin, as caffeine promotes its production. All you actually want from the coffee at this point in your day is a little breathing space, a moment in time just for you. The reasons we crave a hot drink vary, but without realizing it, it is sometimes just to catch our breath. In those coffee-break moments, it is as if there is a bubble around us, and we are silently communicating, "Don't you dare come near me for the next three minutes!" I have had countless women tell me that coffee is the only peace they get in their day, which, if you look at the reality of it, is not true, as physically coffee is actually adding to the demand on the adrenal glands, pushing them to produce adrenalin to get you out of danger that doesn't actually exist.

There is one important difference between the past and the modern-day. The biochemical changes generated by adrenalin, such as sugar being dumped into your blood to get you out of danger, serve a useful purpose when you are physically fighting or fleeing, but if you are sitting at your desk and sugar is dumped into your blood, you make insulin to deal with the elevation in blood sugar. And insulin is one of our primary fat storage hormones. Not only that, but it sets your blood sugar up to crash at a later stage, creating a fatigued state that makes you feel like only more caffeine or high-sugar food can fix it. You can already see how adrenalin might make you go for foods or drinks that you know don't serve your well-being.

HOW COFFEE AMPS YOU UP AND CAN IMPACT ON YOUR SHINE

Over 90 per cent of adults in the Western world consume caffeine daily. More than 50 per cent of Americans consume 13 or more caffeinated drinks per week. In Australia and New Zealand, studies suggest that caffeine consumption has more than tripled since the 1960s and, although levels may not be on par with rates of consumption in the United States, they are rapidly rising, not only due to an increase in coffee consumption but also due to the widespread use of caffeine as an ingredient in, for example, energy drinks. In the United States, 70 per cent of soft drinks contain caffeine. In a US study conducted in 2011, 28 per cent of coffee drinkers had their first cup within 15 minutes of waking and 68 per cent within an hour of waking, while 57 per cent added sugar or sweetener to their brew. The level of caffeine consumption for far too many people is considered addictive by medical textbook standards.

Here's what happens when you consume caffeine.

Caffeine sends a message to the pituitary gland in your brain that it needs to send a message to the adrenal glands to make stress hormones: adrenalin and/or cortisol. When adrenalin is released, your blood sugar elevates to provide you with more energy (fuel); your blood pressure and pulse rate rise to provide more oxygen to the muscles, which tense in preparation for action. Reproductive functions are down-regulated since they use a lot of energy and are not necessary for your immediate survival, given the impending "threat". Plus, your body does not believe it is safe to bring a baby into what it perceives to be an unsafe world, as adrenalin tells your body that your life is in danger and cortisol communicates that there is no more food left in the world!

Adrenalin production can be the result of real or perceived stress, or simply the result of your caffeine intake. Caffeine, via stress hormones, and coupled with the signal to activate the fight-or-flight response, fires you up. Once triggered, in this state you have little hope of being calm, centred, and able to focus on instructions being given to you; for example, by your boss, a colleague, or a receptionist confirming an appointment with you. In addition, this biochemical state puts all of its resources into saving your life rather than into what are considered non-vital processes, processes inside you that nourish skin, hair, nails, and allow the reproductive system to work optimally. Over time, the lack of resources, such as nutrients, available to these so-called non-vital processes has significant consequences internally and externally. First, your skin, hair and nails won't receive the nutrients and other substances they need to look their best. Secondly, because the fuel that drives the fight-or-flight response is glucose ("sugar"), you will crave sugar to constantly refill your fuel tank and you won't utilize your fat stores often or easily. Also, with additional glucose in your blood, you will release insulin — a fat storage hormone — and it will first convert unused glucose from your blood into glycogen and store it in your muscles; what is left over will be converted into body fat.

Let me explain this with the story of a client I'll call Susan.

Susan's Story

This strikingly slim and physically beautiful woman had an appointment to see me. I did what I do with every client, and asked her how I could help and what she would like to get out of our session. Susan apologized for what she thought would sound vain and said that she had gained three kilos (seven pounds) recently and was seeing me because nothing in her diet or activity level had changed and could be attributed to the weight gain. She was concerned that she may be perimenopausal even though her periods had not changed. Some of her friends had gained weight during perimenopause, and she was here because she was concerned that those three kilos would become 10 before she knew it, if she didn't get to the bottom of why her body had changed. I admired Susan's attitude and her desire to understand her body better.

We discussed many facets of her life, emotional and physical, and when it came time to talk about her food, her diet was outstanding with regards to all of my benchmarks for eating a diet based on fresh foods. People like me have numerous strategies that we can apply to assist someone on their quest for body fat loss; from a food perspective, this lady was already living by most of the tricks of my trade. When it came time to talk about her liquid intake, she informed me that she had one glass of red wine four times per week and that she had done this with her husband for years. And then I asked if she drank coffee. Susan's eyes lit up. She replied that, yes, she loved it, but acknowledged, on reflection, that her caffeine intake was something that had changed. She had always had a coffee before breakfast every day for most of her adult life, and that was the only caffeine she consumed all day. But for the past three to four months, she had begun to have up to four coffees per day, but she didn't know why. She just had. When my eyes lit up back at her, she quickly justified her intake by saying, "But they are all black coffees, so there are no calories in them." She drank them all at her desk, she never exercised, and I could see that she had very little muscle mass. Susan herself observed that her fat had gone on around her tummy.

Susan could see from the look on my face where I was about to go and, before I had even spoken, she said "Please don't take them from me." I wanted her to see how emotionally attached she was to this drink so I didn't interrupt her. Eventually, I said that I believed it was the coffee that had led to the change in her body, and she cried. She literally cried. That was impossible, she said, and she kept coming back to the calorie reasoning. Basically, she had a tantrum in my office. I gently tried to lead her to the truth that actually it's only a drink; yet she behaved as though her four daily coffees held the meaning of life for her. I went on to explain the mechanism I have outlined above involving caffeine, adrenalin, elevated blood sugar, and subsequent insulin production. I told her I wasn't even asking her to give up caffeine entirely, but rather go back to her one cup a day before breakfast, a coffee prepared with love by her husband, and see what happened.

Susan agreed to make this change for four weeks, even though she couldn't imagine anything being more powerful than calories in fat creation and couldn't see how this plan could possibly work. I did nothing else for this woman. Not one other change to her dietary intake, and four weeks later she burst through my door telling me she had lost four kilos (nine pounds) in four weeks. She had only gained three (seven pounds) in the first place. As an aside, I have never weighed a client, nor will I ever weigh a client, as I believe you simply weigh your self-esteem when you weigh yourself.

My theory was that Susan's weight gain was the result of stress hormone production from the additional caffeine — and the cascade of effects this can have, including increased insulin release — rather than the result of too many calories. Her subsequent weight loss was, in my opinion, extremely fast, but my point in sharing this story is to demonstrate caffeine's power to signal what is, for some, fat storage, and also its ability to create an almost crazed emotional state, demonstrated by Susan's tantrum when we first. Decreasing her coffee consumption seemed like an overwhelming task for Susan, but she stuck with it and reaped the benefits.

Such fast weight loss will not happen for everyone, but the level of calm and well-being certainly improves with less caffeine. Weight loss significantly depends on the balance between your sympathetic and your parasympathetic nervous systems, which I discuss in detail in my book *Rushing Woman's Syndrome*.

It is so important that you consider your caffeine habits and get honest with yourself about how it affects you. Does it dull your appetite, and so unconsciously you grab a coffee instead of eating? This is especially true for many women at lunchtime. Does it make your heart race, give you the shakes, or loosen your bowels? Does it elevate your blood pressure? Do you notice you want it more when you are stressed and, if so, what story have you attached to what coffee gives you? Do you have restless, poor-quality sleep because of how much caffeine you consume? Does it dull your complexion when you have it daily? Or does it lift your mood or nourish your soul with no ill effect whatsoever? My clients will tell you that, when it is warranted, I ask them to give up caffeine completely for a four-week trial period. They are often shocked by how much more energy they have without caffeine in their lives, not to mention having less or no anxiety! You know yourself better than anyone. Act on what you know is true for you.

Think about all of these mechanisms. So many women run on adrenalin these days. Moment to moment, day to day, it's like a light-switch has gone on, and it hasn't entirely switched off for a really long time. And it doesn't have to be traumatic stress and/or shocking situations that drive this process in us. It can simply be the pace at which we live our lives; being contactable 24/7; constant exposure to social media, unless we purposefully choose otherwise; the juggling act that leads so many women I meet to say that they want more "balance" in their lives, that they can't cope like this anymore, and their perception that their stress is dimming their light. I wrote *Rushing Woman's Syndrome* for women who feel like this and to guide them out of the rush. Have some fun and take the *Rushing Woman's Syndrome* test at: www.drlibby.com/bioresources because resolving the rush can have a significant impact on your health and beauty.

The human body is incredibly resilient and, although we were not designed to withstand long-term stress (due to the way we are designed, we are healthier when it is short-lived), many bodies appear to tolerate, but not necessarily thrive on, years and years of living on adrenalin. Yet I have witnessed first-hand what the relentless production of this hormone does to women's health, including its impact on their fertility, premenstrual syndrome (PMS) and the severity of it, their digestive systems, their skin, their relationships, their happiness, and what I refer to throughout this book as their "shine". It is as if the lights go out in their eyes. An additional challenge, however, is that once the body perceives that the stress has become long-term, your dominant stress hormone can begin to change.

CORTISOL — FRIEND OR WORST NIGHTMARE?

Cortisol is your long-term stress hormone. Historically, the only long-term stress humans had, had revolved around food being scarce. Long-term stress came in the form of floods, famines, and wars. During such times, a person didn't know where the next meal was coming from. Today, in the Western world, our long-term stresses tend to be based more on financial situations, relationship concerns, challenges with friendships, particularly for teenage girls, and uncertainty or worries about your health or body. I can't tell you how many times I have heard women say they would "do anything" for a different body part — thinner thighs, less body hair, no cellulite — and for many women the part or parts of themselves that they dislike intensely become a silent fixation of worry in their minds. For so many women, their first waking thoughts involve "What will I or won't I eat today?" or "How much exercise can I get done today?"

So many women rush through their days with a pervasive not-good-enough or never-enough-time monologue running through their head. Day after day, this can easily lead to a chronic pattern of stress response, hence increased cortisol output. In turn, this can lead to a change in your metabolism, and essentially your behaviour, because while you feel like you can't keep up, your body's perception is that it has to do everything at a rapid pace. Unfortunately, biochemically this all takes away from your body's ability to rest, restore, replenish, and revitalize the "beauty bits", because your body thinks, "Why on Earth would I take care of her skin, hair, and nails, when there's a famine going on?" Your body's perception is that it is doing you a great big favour by putting all of its resources toward saving your life.

How Cortisol Works

It is important to understand how cortisol works, as it can be your friend or one of your worst nightmares. When made at optimum amounts, cortisol does numerous wonderful things for your health. It is one of the body's primary anti-inflammatory mediators, meaning that wherever there is inflammation in the body, cortisol, having been converted into cortisone, dampens down the effect of that inflammation and stops your body from feeling stiff, rigid, or in pain. Many people, for example, describe feeling that they have suddenly aged as they come out of difficult times, and often this is the result of suboptimal cortisol levels during such periods. In the right amount, cortisol is not only an anti-inflammatory, it also buffers the effect of insulin, meaning that optimum amounts help you continue to burn body fat for energy while also maintaining stable (as opposed to rapidly fluctuating) blood sugar levels.

Cortisol levels change over the day. The right amount at the right time assists you with various bodily functions throughout the course of the day. Cortisol is designed to be high in the morning and, for the purpose of this discussion, let's say that 25 units at around 6am is ideal. Cortisol is one of the mechanisms that wake you up in the morning and help you bounce out of bed full of energy and vitality, rather than snooze an hour away. By midday, optimum cortisol will sit at around 15 units and, by 6pm, levels will ideally be at around four units. By 10pm, optimum cortisol levels are around two units, a level at which they are designed to stay until around 2am, when they slowly and very steadily begin to rise again.

The following graph illustrates this. So it is true what your mother told you — that one hour of sleep before midnight is worth two after — because cortisol starts to rise around 2am and the waking-up process gradually begins.

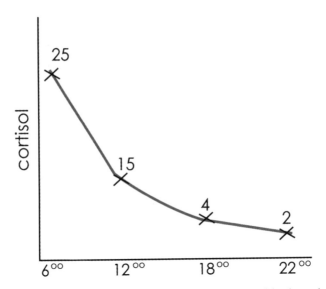

The optimal cortisol profile: Cortisol is nice and high in the morning, and falls away again by the evening.

As a stress response continues, its effect on the body begins to change. In the early stages of stress, one of the first challenges cortisol presents is that the evening level of the hormone starts to spike again rather than continue to decrease. At this stage, you still make optimum levels in the morning and are able to bounce out of bed and get on with your day with reasonable energy, but evening levels are creeping up. This is one mechanism through which good sleeping patterns can be interrupted. We all know that sleep is a critical beauty foundation for so many reasons, which is why it has a chapter all of its own.

When cortisol levels become elevated above optimal, other changes in body chemistry begin to unfold. It has been suggested that elevated cortisol is the one common thread behind what we have come to describe as metabolic syndrome; that is, elevated blood pressure, elevated cholesterol, and insulin resistance. This last condition is a warning sign that, if nothing changes in the near future, type 2 diabetes is a likely consequence. If we remember that we are completely geared for survival, and that elevated cortisol tells every cell of our body that food is scarce, another of its roles is to slow down your metabolic rate. A slower metabolism leads you to burn body fat for energy far more slowly than you have in the past, as cortisol is designed to make sure that you survive this perceived period of famine.

Cortisol is "catabolic", meaning that it breaks protein down into its building blocks, known as amino acids. This catabolism is one of the mechanisms through which cortisol slows your metabolism. Your muscles are made from proteins, and cortisol signals them to break down, as the body's perception is that fuel is needed. Additional amino acids are also needed in the blood to help repair tissues, even though you may be simply sitting on your bottom in front of the television, with your financial or relationship concerns milling around in your head! The amino acids released as a result of the catabolic signalling of cortisol can be converted, through a process called "gluconeogenesis", back into glucose (sugar), which your body thinks may be useful to assist you in your stress. Yet, if you are not active, this increase in blood glucose will not be utilized, and insulin will have to be secreted to return blood glucose levels to normal by returning the glucose in the blood to storage. Remember that glucose is stored as glycogen in the muscles and the liver.

Over time, the catabolic signalling of cortisol itself may have broken down some of your muscles, so now there is less space for glucose storage. As a result, some of the blood glucose returns to the remaining muscles while the leftovers are converted into body fat. Keeping the glucose level of the blood within the normal, safe range is of more importance to your body than whether you have wobbly bits around your middle! Essentially, too much cortisol can make you fat through dysregulated blood sugar metabolism, not just fat metabolism itself. This is one of the mechanisms through which cellulite can appear (we will explore some others and what you can do about it later), as where muscles once were, fat can now be deposited. This is also the process through which long-term stress can lead to type 2 diabetes.

Because excess cortisol is produced after the stress in your life has been going on for a while, your body — not knowing any better — thinks there is no more food left in your world, and it instinctively knows that it has a greater chance of survival if it holds on to some extra body fat. In modern times, when, for health reasons or vanity (or both), many people understand the importance of not carrying too much body fat, cortisol can provide a potential challenge to someone who believes that eating less is their only solution to body fat loss. Yet if you eat less when excess cortisol is already telling your body that there is no food left in the world, you will confirm that belief and your metabolism will be slowed even further. Feeling like she is fighting an uphill battle with her body can be an immense source of stress for a woman, adding another layer of stress to an already busy life.

Understanding the Cortisol Problem

If cortisol tells every cell of your body that food is scarce, and your metabolism slows down as a result, and you continue to eat and exercise in the same way you always have, your clothes will slowly get tighter. It doesn't matter how amazingly you eat; with cortisol telling every cell in your body to store fat, it is very difficult, if not impossible, to decrease body fat until the cortisol issue is resolved. We must get to the heart of the stress and either change the situation or change the perception. That doesn't mean you give up on taking care of how you nourish your body, though! It needs all of the nutrients it can get, even more so when there is stress. Just remember that focusing on the calorie equation — how much you eat versus how much you move — won't solve a waistline that is expanding due to elevated cortisol.

Cortisol has a distinct fat deposition pattern. If cortisol is an issue for you, you typically lay it on around your tummy and, once again, the reason for fat placement here is governed by the body's quest for survival. If food suddenly did run out, your major organs have easy access to fat that will keep you alive. You also tend to lay fat down on the back of the arms (you get "bingo wings"), and you grow what I lovingly call a back veranda. So what do most people do when they notice that their clothes are getting tighter? They go on a diet, which typically means eating less. Eating less, though, just confirms to your body what it perceives to be true — that food is scarce — and that slows down your metabolism even further. But food is not scarce; it is abundant for you. If you want a chocolate bar at 3am, you can get one.

Another challenge you face with elevated cortisol is that, since your body thinks that food is scarce, any time you see food it is very easy to over-eat. No matter how firmly you intend to eat only three crackers when you get home from work, if that open packet of crackers is in front of you, cortisol will scream at every cell of your body: "You are so lucky! There's food here — eat it!" And somehow, before you know it, the whole box of crackers is gone. Don't get me wrong: I am not saying that self-discipline and willpower have no place. You could make a decision right now that when it comes to what you put into your body, from this point forward you are going to raise your standards. You could do that right now. My intention in explaining this is simply to point out that humans have very ancient hormonal mechanisms at work inside their bodies that believe they know better than you when it comes to your survival. Your body can be your biggest teacher if you learn how to decipher its messages. Extra body fat, congested skin, and/or whichever body part you focus on and wish you could change, are sometimes simply vehicles of communication, asking you to explore your biochemistry and your beliefs that have led to this situation.

SILENT STRESS

What about when the stress is silent? You might not be a drama queen running around, arms flailing all over the place, screeching "I'm so stressed, I'm so stressed!" You may be a private person and keep things mostly to yourself. You may be so private with your fears and concerns, always presenting a happy face to the world, that you don't even realize that you are worried about things or recognize that you may have been in a stressed state for a very long time. You are like the boiling frog …

There is a wonderful analogy I use to describe how people have become oblivious to the stress and pressure in their lives. It is about a frog, and, since green tree frogs just happen to be one of my favourite creatures on the planet, and one of my nicknames is Frog, it appeals to me even more! If you put a frog in cool water, it swims around very happily. If you put a frog in boiling water, it immediately jumps out to save itself. But if you put a frog in cool water and slowly bring that water to the boil, the frog doesn't notice and doesn't jump out.

I believe that most people in the Western world would jump out of the pressure in their lives if they were suddenly thrown into it. But we don't jump out when it gradually increases over the years. We don't tend to notice until a crisis hits — the death of someone we love or our own health crashes. Don't let it take a health crisis to wake you up to the fact that without your health you have nothing. If you see in yourself the frog whose world has slowly been on the boil, act now to change it. Begin to put in place strategies to either change your situation or your perception of your life, or both. This book will cover many options open to you. Either way, the changes you can foster in your biochemistry, your emotional landscape, and as a result your overall well-being, are potentially enormous.

Guilt and Cortisol

When you feel grateful for the life you have, it is easy to feel guilty if you complain about anything. A common internal phrase might be "There are so many people worse off than me." Such thinking immediately makes you feel guilty, and you stop focusing on your source of stress. Trouble is, although there *are* people worse off than you in this world, the minute you feel guilty you change your focus so that you don't ever get the opportunity to truly identify what is bothering you, and more importantly why.

Many women keep the peace to avoid stress. Yet there is no peace when you have to keep the peace. Here's a common example to help you see how everyday life, because of the perceptions we bring to it, can lead to cortisol, from an emotional source, being a contributor to your health and beauty challenges.

Basic psychology teaches us that humans will do more to avoid pain than they will ever do to experience pleasure. Some women I meet will do anything, for example, to keep the peace and avoid conflict. Inwardly, they become highly strung because they are always walking on eggshells around others, especially their intimate partner, doing all they can to help prevent those around them from losing their temper. If the man of the house has a tendency to communicate with explosive, angry outbursts that seem unpredictable, well hello silent stress hormone production!

Some women avoid feeling emotional pain by eating too much or making other poor food choices; perhaps drinking bucket-loads of wine or chain-smoking cigarettes. Some go shopping and rack up credit card bills that will take months or years to pay. Alternatively, some people might cope or explore their pain by writing in a journal, going for a walk, a run, or a swim. Others will pray, meditate, or telephone a friend and chat to deal with emotional pain. Some of the ways we cope with or explore what is going on support our health. Some potentially harm our health. And all of these activities may take place with or without a conscious understanding of why.

I want to help you see *why*, so that you can change your response, if it is hurting your health, especially if the stress hormone production triggered by your subconscious emotional responses is blocking you from experiencing the shining light that you are.

WORRYING IS NO GOOD FOR YOUR HEALTH

As we now know, stress — whether it is real or perceived — may promote the production of excess cortisol. The ripple effect of a worry can slowly and subtly change your metabolism to one of fat storage, leave your headspace full of sadness, and cause you to withdraw. For some, worry is at the heart of why they no longer feel like they shine as they once did. And what is driving this are the chemical signals created by your body, which it believes will help you based on the information it is receiving.

You think you want to lose weight more than anything? You think you would do anything to be slimmer? You probably already have all of the healthy eating information you need to do this. So, what's stopping you? Or what stops you once you have started? On the flip side, maybe you eat too little, or binge and then purge, or perhaps you just punish yourself mentally for everything you eat that you don't consider to be "healthy". Whatever the scenario, you know on some level that the way you eat, or don't eat, is harming you, yet you don't make a change in this area of your life. The example below is of over-eating, but if under-eating applies to you, replace the over-eating concepts with under-eating. The message is the same either way: you don't know why you do what you do when you know what you know.

Every day of my working life, I meet people who eat too much. They know they do, but they can't seem to stop. Sometimes it is nutritious food, sometimes it is not, but, whatever the case, they know they would be much better off if they ate less. Often these people are seeing me because they want to lose weight, and they are precious, intelligent people who don't understand why they do what they do. These people know what to eat and what not to eat to lose weight, yet they don't do it, even though they truly believe that they are desperate to lose weight.

There is a really big difference between eating two squares of chocolate and eating the entire block, between one biscuit (cookie) with a cup of tea in the evening and a dozen. We all know that eating too much makes us feel full and uncomfortable, but, worse, it usually drives us to say very unkind things to ourselves such as "I'm so useless, I have no willpower", and leads us to go to bed feeling guilty and sad and believing we will never be able to change. The belief that things are permanent is destructive.

So what might be going on for someone who, even with good intentions, just can't stop eating? Besides elevated cortisol caused by long-term stress, there may be other biochemical factors involved, such as low progesterone, poor thyroid function, or blood sugar that surges and plummets, as explored in later chapters. There are also likely to be emotional factors and core beliefs that they probably aren't even aware of. Everyone has a different *why*. I want to help you find yours so you can tend to it and let your light grow.

ADRENAL FATIGUE

The next biochemical stage of stress that can occur, especially if the stress has been prolonged, may involve cortisol falling low, and I see more and more of this in younger and younger women these days. If you have had a high level of cortisol output for many, many years, your adrenal glands may not be able to stand the tension. They are not designed to sustain this kind of output, and so they crash. In general terms, you burn out. Your light fizzles. In more recent times, this has become known as adrenal fatigue, because the major symptom is a deep, unrelenting fatigue. Yet even with fatigue as the major symptom, what I have observed over the past decade is that not only are women beyond tired, at the same time they can also be wired. And when you are tired but wired, you desire deeply restorative sleep more than ever, yet it rarely happens; your adrenal hormone production is usually at the heart of this. Remember that the pituitary gland is the master switch, and, although treatment for adrenal fatigue usually involves a range of strategies that support the adrenals themselves, going one step further and assisting the pituitary gland can also be immensely powerful and highly beneficial to restoring your health and vitality.

As you now understand, the adrenal hormone cortisol is supposed to be high in the morning, helping you to bounce out of bed. It plays a role in how vital you feel and helps the body combat any inflammatory processes that want to kick in. Stiffness is a key symptom of adrenal fatigue. For those with chronic stress, morning cortisol levels tend to be low; if 25 units is the ideal, with adrenal stress you may only get to 10 units. It can be very difficult to get out of bed with such low levels. By mid-afternoon it will be at an all-time low, and you feel you need something sweet, something containing caffeine, or a nap to get you through your afternoon. (This can also be the result of low blood sugar or poor thyroid function, explored in a later section.) For an adrenally fatigued person, cortisol is nice and low in the evenings, as it is supposed to be. But, if you don't go to bed before 10pm, you will typically get a second wind, and it will be much harder for you to fall asleep if you are still up at midnight, partly due to the body's natural next adrenalin (not cortisol) surge that tends to happen between 10.30pm and 11.30pm. The following graph illustrates this cortisol pattern.

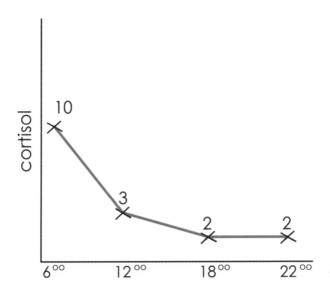

A typical cortisol profile of an adrenally fatigued person: Note, particularly, the low waking cortisol and low midday reading.

When cortisol drops low, it is likely that prior to this it was high (although not always) and body fat may have increased during this time. But just because cortisol is low does not necessarily mean easy access to body fat burning, due to cortisol's relationship to insulin, as described earlier.

Additionally, the fatigue you feel with this biochemical picture may make exercise the least appealing thing on the planet to you. You actually feel worse after cardiovascular exercise when you are adrenally fatigued, whereas exercise typically energizes. Frustration mounts because, like most people in the Western world, you probably believe that exercising and eating less are the only solutions to weight loss, yet you can't bring yourself to do either despite every good intention. You eat something sweet, or consume highly processed carbs in desperate search of energy, or you eat too much, or another month goes past without much movement … When you reflect on this, you feel guilty, you might say mean things to yourself, and you may silently lose hope. Your clothes keep getting tighter, and this just adds to your stress. You can see how this vicious cycle can be self-perpetuating.

Humans were never designed to sustain long-term stress, and our individual bodies cope with it in different ways. For some, adrenalin remains the dominant stress hormone all of their lives, while others may flip over into a more cortisol-dominant stress response. If the stress response doesn't truly switch off, there is the potential that the adrenals will eventually crash, and cortisol output is no longer optimum or elevated. It will be negligible. At its extreme, this can become a condition called Addison's disease. Yet if a person's cortisol level is extremely low but still falls just inside the "normal range", they will be told that they are fine. They may feel lousy, but all the tests they have always come back "normal". They feel anything but normal, and people who know and love them will often comment that they are a shell of their former selves.

Cortisol can also be rather sinister in that it can interfere with your steroid (sex) hormone metabolism;

your sleep patterns, via its interference with mela-tonin; and also your mood, via serotonin — all elements we will look at as we continue.

The Importance of Perceptions

Our perceptions play an enormous role in whether we are stressed or not. Sometimes trauma in the past takes a toll on your well-being: while in your mind you have dealt with it or moved on, your subconscious mind is still wrestling with it. Or stress can be from comparatively minor things. It is as if you have an itch that somehow gets scratched by your beloved, your children, your boss, or by random people. Our bodies go through everything with us, and, despite our minds consciously moving on, sometimes our bodies seem stuck in the past. The messages on these pages will allow you to open yourself up to a new perspective on health, food, movement, life, feeling, and your beliefs, and thereby feel calm and safe, as well as help you understand how each one affects your shine. There are some wonderful methods through which you can help shift your body and your emotions when you feel like you have cognitively processed your stress, yet it still remains a challenge, your weight is still stuck, or you overreact to the undulations of life, where once you were more easily able to laugh at the calamity, the chaos, and the small stuff.

The Importance of Rest

You will see from both the Beautiful Sleep and the Beautiful Solutions chapters later in the book that at the heart of all of my strategies to support you adrenally is the desire for you to rest and to rest well, in a restorative and revitalizing way. Rest must follow action for us to have optimal health, excellent fat burning, the ability to remain calm, and all those "non-vital" processes mentioned earlier, such as our skin, hair, and nails getting all the nourishment they need. And very few of us these days truly rest or live a calm state, where productivity, patience, and kindness tend to easily flow.

In *Rushing Woman's Syndrome*, I talk at length about the nervous system. But, for now, all I need you to understand is that there is a part of our nervous system, the parasympathetic nervous system (PNS), which is active when we truly rest. This is also called the "rest, digest, repair, reproduce" (and I've added "radiance") arm of our nervous system. I also refer to it as the "green zone". The challenge is that it can be dominated by the opposite arm of the nervous system, the sympathetic nervous system (SNS), which I refer to as the "red zone".

Appropriate activation of the PNS is essential not only to our feeling centred, calm, and lovely, but also to a tummy that isn't bloated after eating. Food is not supposed to bloat us, yet a bloated stomach is a major complaint of more than 70 per cent of women in the Western world. Calm is vital to optimal digestion. I have received countless emails from women who have taken my advice to focus on chewing well, on eating slowly, and on eating more real food), who, after even three days, no longer bloat. Imagine that. This happens because:

- eating like this, instead of inhaling food, slows down, or stops, stress hormone production, allowing the blood supply to support the digestive system

- chewing food well stimulates stomach acid and digestive enzymes, enhancing digestion

- the body knows how to digest real food.

The Importance of Diaphragmatic Breathing

Breathing is the only way we can consciously affect our autonomic nervous system (ANS), the part of the nervous system from where the red and green zones stem. We cannot control our ANS with our thoughts; we cannot instruct it what to do. How we breathe is our only road in there. Every time I write or say that out loud, I am reminded of just how magical and miraculous the human body is.

The impact of diaphragmatic breathing on the nervous system is one of the main reasons why it is the cornerstone of all my adrenal support solutions. If you take nothing else away from this book, I would like to encourage you with every ounce of my being to incorporate a ritual into your day that allows you to focus on breathing well. It is not only key to shifting our chemistry from fat storage to fat burning and for cultivating calm, but it is also the most crucial strategy for feeling like we shine. How can the breath drive such powerful shifts in your nervous system and your biochemistry?

The role of the ANS is to perceive the external environment and, after processing the information in the central nervous system, regulate the function of your internal environment. The name "autonomic" implies that it is independent of the conscious mind. Think about a family of ducks and their newborn ducklings. Just like ducklings, the autonomic nervous system will always follow the leader, and the breath is the *only* part of the autonomic nervous system that can be controlled consciously. Your breath leads. Your body follows. Breathing dominates your autonomic nervous system, and because we breathe 5000 to 30,000 times a day — or 200 million to 500 million times in a lifetime — it has the potential to influence us positively, or negatively, in many ways.

Nothing communicates to every cell of your body that you are safe better than your breathing. If you breathe in a shallow way, with short, sharp inhalations and exhalations, then you are communicating that your life is in danger. Remember the cascade of hormonal events that follow such an alarm, and the role these hormones play, for one thing, in switching fat burning on or off. How you breathe is also a fast-track to the symptoms of anxiety, and potentially panic attacks, regardless of what led you to breathe in a shallow way in the first place. Whether it was an event, a deadline, the perception of pressure, the "need" to rush, or the lifetime habit of your nervous system, the result is the same. Long, slow breathing that moves your diaphragm communicates the opposite message to your body — that you are very safe. Nothing down-regulates the production of fat storage stress hormones or the alarm signals within your body more powerfully. No practice restores your vitality like regularly breathing this way. And I don't say that lightly.

Practise diaphragmatic breathing, making sure your tummy moves in and out as you breathe, as opposed to just your upper chest. You can begin your breath by allowing the lower part of your tummy to expand, and then imagine as the breath slowly continues that the expansion of your tummy has now extended into the area where you can feel your ribcage meet. Keep the slow inhalation going until your upper chest feels like it is pushing your ribs out at the sides of your body. Then pause, rather than hold your breath, and slowly allow the exhalation to begin in the reverse order of the inhalation, with the top and side of the chest emptying first, followed by the middle of your abdomen and lastly your tummy. If that sounds or feels too tricky, just move your tummy (abdomen) in and out with each breath, allow it to expand on the inhale and shrink back on the exhale.

Be kind and patient with yourself, as this takes practice! You may feel like you are unable to get parts of your body to engage at first, but in time and with practice the parts of you that have become disconnected will be thrilled to be back in touch.

At first, you will more than likely need to schedule regular breathing time slots into your day until it becomes your new way of breathing. Make appointments with yourself to breathe. If it is peaceful each morning while you boil the kettle for the first time that day (to make your hot water with lemon, of course), instead of racing around and doing 80 jobs while the kettle boils, stand in your kitchen and breathe. Link breathing well to a daily routine, such as having a shower, or to a particular hour of the day so that it quickly becomes a habit. Do it numerous times over the course of your day. Book a meeting into your calendar each afternoon at 3pm. If you work at a computer, have it pop up on the screen that it is time for your meeting with yourself to do 20 long, slow breaths. We keep appointments with other people, so be sure to keep the appointments you make with yourself. Take part in movement that facilitates a focus on the breath such as t'ai chi, qigong, yoga, particularly restorative yoga, or walking quietly in Nature. Pilates can also be useful, but I have found that it is highly dependent on your attitude while you are doing the session, and also to some degree on the attitude of the instructor. For me personally, qigong is how I choose to begin my day. It is not always easy to make happen, but it is my habit now and has been for years. I had a period of time where I let this ritual go, and I soon learnt how crucial it is to set up my day with a restoration-focused session. Without it, my clarity, my sex hormone balance, and my vitality are not what I know they can be. So, please, schedule breathing-focused periods into your day, and keep your appointments with yourself. Breathing is the cornerstone of calm, and therefore of optimal health and beauty from the inside out, and these practices allow us to still the stories that for many women fill their minds and are part of their source of stress.

The Importance of Laughter

Another free and powerful tool is laughter. If we see life as tough, and full of hard work, pain, and drudgery, it will be precisely that. Humans have the ability to only see their perspective in the world, rather than the world as it truly is. We see the world through filters, even though we don't know they are there. I am not denying that life can be tough at times, or that being honest with ourselves if we do feel down and out about life is not a good thing. The problem comes when we see the world this way and believe that it will never be any different. For then it won't be.

Think about it. A belief in the permanence of doom is dangerous for every hormonal signal in your body. Do your absolute best to shift your thinking to see life as an adventure, a journey, a gift full of opportunity, and a process through which you can contribute. Some of the greatest, most moving stories I have ever heard involved someone turning a horrific hardship into their greatest opportunity. Keep this in mind. Keep in mind, too, that you can choose to laugh at the calamity around you. I remember clearly witnessing this when my dearest friend had her third baby, and, with him not even a day old, countless well-wishers chattering away, a hospital staff member wanting to clear the food tray away, and her deliciously spirited two-year-old daughter not being too thrilled about this as she wanted the remaining apple juice — and all in one small room — my precious friend and her husband just shrugged and grinned at each other and laughed, internally clearly focused on the love in the room, rather than on anything else. What you focus on is what you feel.

The influence of a beautiful, helpful, hopeful character is contagious. People radiate what is in their minds and in their hearts.

Eleanor H. Porter

Chapter 4
Part 2

Beautiful Sex Hormones:
the role of their balance in your beauty

Another system intimately involved in whether we feel like we have got our sparkle on or not, and in our capacity to feel calm, cope, and be happy involves the various glands and tissues that produce our sex hormones. In females, the ovaries are the main source of sex hormone production; however, both the adrenal glands and fat cells make sex hormones, too. The body also contains tissues that produce hormones themselves, but are not sensitive to hormone levels in our body. The reason some tissues are hormone-sensitive and some are not relates to the presence of receptors for a particular hormone being present on that tissue. Let me explain.

HORMONES AND RECEPTORS: LIKE LOCKS AND KEYS

Just because your body makes a certain hormone, that doesn't mean you get the lovely or the not-so-lovely effects of the hormone. For a hormone to illicit its effects, it has to bind to a receptor. The best way to imagine the way hormones interact with a receptor site is like a lock and a key. When they connect, you get the effects of the hormone. Breast tissue, for example, is highly sensitive to oestrogen and progesterone, the two main female sex hormones, because the breasts contain receptors for both of these hormones.

Sex hormones can be delicious substances that give you energy and vitality, and yet they can also wreak havoc on your life. When it comes to a sense of calm, mental clarity, the ability to be patient and not make mountains out of molehills, fat burning, beautiful skin, as well as fertility, very few substances in our body impact us more than our sex hormones.

The main sex hormones we will cover are oestrogen, progesterone, and testosterone, with a particular focus on their role in body shape, size, fat burning, inner peace, and outward sparkle; for when sex hormones are out of balance, this alone can leave you feeling all pent-up or utterly spent and bedraggled.

Oestrogen is a feminine hormone (although men naturally make it in small amounts), and it plays numerous important roles in the human body, including ones associated with reproduction, new bone growth, and cardiovascular health. Challenges with oestrogen occur, however, when there is too much of it compared to other hormones, progesterone in particular. Oestrogen can also pose a problem if there is too much of one type of oestrogen compared to other types of oestrogen.

The ovaries of menstruating females make oestrogen, and small amounts are produced by fat cells and the adrenal glands. At menopause, ovarian production of hormones ceases.

From a reproductive perspective, oestrogen's role in the female body is to lay down the lining of the uterus, which it does between days 1 and 14 of a typical 28-day reproductive cycle, with day 1 of the cycle being the first day of menstruation. The oestrogen lays the lining of the uterus down over these first 14 days to prepare the female body for a conception if it takes place. Oestrogen wants a menstruating female to fall pregnant every single month of her life — whether that is on her agenda or not! Remember, our bodies are completely geared for survival, and perpetuation of the human species is an enormous part of that survival process.

As a result of the biological imperative to conceive each month, oestrogen ensures there is adequate body fat, as most females do not immediately know that they are pregnant. In the event that the woman is a stick figure without much body fat, it is possible that a brand-new foetus may not survive. To prevent this, oestrogen signals fat to be laid down in typically female areas, giving women a pear-like shape to better serve the childbirth process.

Oestrogen is the hormone that makes female breasts bud at the first signs of puberty, it broadens hips, and gives women their curves. It lays down fat on a woman's hips, bottom, and thighs, and is typically responsible for making the bottom half of a female body broader than the top half. Oestrogen also, unfortunately, promotes fluid retention when it is in excess, and this alone can be very stressful for a female. Her clothes don't fit her the way she would like them to, and the last thing she wants when she feels "puffy and swollen" is to be intimate, which for some women can lead to challenges with their significant other. This can add another layer of stress to what may feel like an already overwhelming life.

Fluid Retention

I am convinced that many women feel fat when really they are either bloated or retaining fluid. As I said earlier, I never weigh clients and I don't encourage them to weigh themselves. I do this for many reasons, but one is that as hormone levels fluctuate over the month so can the amounts of fluid being retained, until the hormones return to balance. Besides, when you weigh yourself, remember that all you are really weighing is your self-esteem. I have met thousands of women who can gain three kilos (six pounds) in a day — to say that this messes with their minds is an understatement. If you get on the scales in the morning and weigh 70 kilograms (155 pounds), and by the evening you weigh 73 kilograms (161 pounds), especially if you have eaten well and exercised that day, and even if you *haven't* eaten well or exercised that day, it is easy to feel incredibly disheartened and wonder how on Earth this could possibly happen. Weight can feel like just another thing to worry and panic about, which does little to help with your glow.

Remember this: it is not physically possible to gain three kilos (six pounds) of body fat in a single day. The only possible cause is fluid retention. Yet, even though the logical part of the female mind knows this, seeing three extra kilos on the scales over the course of just a day, or even a week, will make most women, no matter how reasonable they are, feel fat, anxious, impatient, frustrated, and generally lousy. And are you more likely to make good food choices when you feel this way? Are you likely to want to be intimate with your partner when you feel fleshy and puffy and as though there is not enough time in your day, because you are eating well and exercising and still gaining weight? When you think that this must mean you have to find the time to do even more exercise, and you don't know where on Earth that time is going to come from because you already can't keep up — and that was all thought in such a hurry that by now you are gulping for air!

There can be numerous factors behind fluid retention — too many to go into here — but, in a nutshell, fluid retention can be driven by poor lymphatic flow, a congested liver from too many liver loaders, mineral deficiencies and imbalances, and poor progesterone production. From an energetic medicine perspective, I also encourage you to think about who or what you may be holding onto that no longer benefits you. Perhaps it is a belief that no longer serves you, and your body is simply trying to wake you up to this and get you to change. So many of us fear change whether we realize it or not.

Excess oestrogen can be another likely culprit when it comes to fluid retention. It can also drive headaches, including migraines, increase blood clotting, decrease libido, interfere with thyroid hormone production, and, due to its relationship with progesterone, lead us to feel like we have to do everything with haste. So, big health and therefore beauty consequences all because there is too much of one little hormone.

Progesterone plays a variety of roles in the human body. From a reproductive perspective, its job is to hold in place the lining of the uterus that oestrogen lays down between days 1 and 14 of your cycle. If your body detects that a conception has taken place, the lining of the uterus needs to be maintained and thickened, rather than shed. As a result, progesterone levels begin to rise. If there is no conception, the lining of the uterus is not needed, and progesterone levels fall away, which initiates menstruation. When health is optimal, progesterone is the dominant sex hormone from just after mid-cycle until menstruation.

Biologically, progesterone has numerous other roles, all pivotal to the *Beauty from the Inside Out* message. Progesterone is a powerful anti-anxiety agent, an antidepressant, and a diuretic, and it is essential if you are to access fat reserves to burn for energy. Without the right amounts of progesterone, you will always burn your sugar, which may lead to your body having to break down your muscles for energy rather than accessing and burning fat stores; this, over time, slows your metabolic rate. You may also have a tendency towards an anxious or depressed mood — and if you feel like you have a blessed life and yet you still feel flat, add guilt to that emotional cocktail and a degree of confusion about what is really bothering you. You can see how layer upon layer of physical and emotional stress can form, which is a sure-fire way for women to feel like their sparkle has diminished ... or even been extinguished.

THE RELATIONSHIP BETWEEN STRESS AND SEX HORMONES

The relationship between sex hormones and stress hormones is fascinating and powerful, and it is where an aspect of the physical, biochemical approach of *Beauty from the Inside Out* is focused. This is because 9 out of 10 women who see me for consultations enjoy positive changes in their body and their well-being when we address this.

Oestrogen is the dominant sex hormone between day 1 and day 14 of the menstrual cycle. For the first half of the menstrual cycle, a relatively small amount of progesterone is made from the adrenal glands. For the sake of this description, let's call the amount two units. Remember, the reproductive role of progesterone is to hold in place the lining of the uterus, with the additional biological functions of it being an anti-anxiety agent, an antidepressant, and a diuretic. Optimal levels of progesterone are highly linked to you getting your glow on, so you want to support your body's natural production (covered in the Beautiful Solutions chapter).

However, as you now understand, your adrenal glands are also where you make your stress hormones, namely adrenalin and cortisol. Adrenalin communicates to every cell of your body that your life is being threatened, even though all you may have done is had an argument with your beloved, and he spoke to you inappropriately because he felt like a failure at the time. Men usually don't behave well when they subconsciously create a meaning of failure from something that's happened, which could come from a question you asked (without any loaded meaning behind it), or because he looked his bank balance earlier that day and it is not where he needs it to be to feel safe. Women typically behave in a way they, or those around them, don't enjoy so much when they feel rejected, unloved, or unappreciated. This does not excuse poor behaviour, but rather offers an explanation to promote understanding. My point is to highlight that both physical (for example, caffeine) and emotional (for example, a perception of pressure or creating a meaning of rejection from an argument) processes can drive adrenalin production and communicate that danger is present.

As you now understand, when you are internally rattled, cortisol communicates to every cell in your body that there is no food left in the world, and as a result it wants your body to break down muscle and store fat. Even though food is abundant for you, and your cortisol production is likely to be coming from areas of your life about which you feel uncertain — such as relationships, finances, or even what others might think of you — your body thinks there must be a flood, famine, or war, as historically these were the only sources of long-term stress that humans experienced.

Since your body links progesterone to fertility, if your body perceives that your life is under threat and that there is no food left in the world, the last thing it wants is for you to conceive, so it thinks it is doing you a great big favour by shutting down the adrenal production of progesterone. Oestrogen and cortisol, both signalling fat storage and ongoing stress, remain, while you have lost the counterbalancing hormone that keeps you calm and not anxious, and helps burn fat and get rid of excess fluid. Think about it.

I believe this situation alone is a modern-day, monumental shift in female chemistry, and it can torment a woman's emotional and physical well-being. This shift plays an enormous role in whether you feel like you sparkle or you drag yourself through each day, and why you might feel a need to do everything with urgency. A female can go from feeling happy, healthy, balanced, and energized, with great clarity of mind and an even mood, to having a foggy brain and feeling either overly anxious about things she cannot name, or utterly exhausted, as a result of this shift to constant stress hormone production and the subsequent low level (or absence) of progesterone. Physically, she may feel puffy, heavy, bloated, and full of fluid, with a sense that her clothes are getting tighter by the minute (whether this is actually true or not). And that is just the first half of the cycle!

A menstruating female ovulates around day 14 of her cycle, and there are numerous hormonal changes that occur to drive ovulation. Once the egg has been released from the ovary, a crater remains on the surface of the ovary where the egg popped out. This crater is called the corpus luteum, and this is where the bulk of a woman's progesterone is generated. Progesterone is designed to peak on day 21 of a 28-day cycle, at around 25 to 40 units. If conception takes place, progesterone levels need to climb to continue to hold the lining of the uterus in place. Once the placenta has formed by week 12 of gestation, progesterone levels climb to around 300 to 400 units. Pregnancy is the time when a woman has the highest level of circulating progesterone, which is why many women glow, especially from the second trimester onwards. Once a woman has birthed the placenta, however, her progesterone level plunges from 350 to zero! It is fortunate that birth brings on some other feel good hormones, such as oxytocin, although they tend to be more short-lived.

Historically, babies were welcomed into extended families and communities. Today, a more common scenario (not the only scenario) is a hospital birth followed by a new mother at home alone with her newborn during the day while her partner must continue to work to pay the mortgage and other bills. If there are challenges in their relationship, or challenges caused by the needs of other children, financial stress, ill or aging parents, an ill newborn or simply one who won't sleep, the new home environment with baby can be highly stressful. Another common stressful scenario is one where a new mother has made what she thought would be a welcome transition (temporarily or permanently) from a corporate career to staying at home with her baby, but is now second-guessing her decision. The guilt and confusion around this scenario can be overwhelming. Such scenarios do not promote the restoration of adrenal progesterone levels, as the body is so busy making stress hormones that it is not "safe" for the new mum to make the fertility-linked progesterone. Remember, progesterone is one of the most powerful anti-anxiety and antidepressant substances the body makes. On the other hand, if mum and baby do have support, and the new mum doesn't feel she is alone with her new precious bundle — whether this is simply due to the mother's beliefs, attitudes, and perceptions, or her actual physical support from other people — then adrenal progesterone levels are far more likely to be restored, and her chemistry is all the better for it.

If conception does not take place during a menstrual cycle, maintaining the lining of the uterus is no longer necessary and progesterone levels fall, allowing a female to bleed. However, something that is common today is "luteal phase insufficiency", where ovarian progesterone production is poor and the peak of 25 units in the second half of the cycle is not reached. In this situation, progesterone may be the dominant hormone from day 16 to day 18 of the cycle, but it falls away too soon (it is supposed to be dominant from just after mid-cycle until around day 27), and oestrogen becomes dominant leading into the menstrual bleed.

This oestrogen dominance is the biochemical basis of premenstrual syndrome (PMS), which causes grief for the woman as well as for most people around her! When PMS occurs, it can be because oestrogen is dominant for all but two or three days of a 28-day cycle, meaning that progesterone gets very little, if any time to rule the roost, and a woman misses out on all its delicious stress-busting and shine-inducing qualities.

When Oestrogen is Dominant

Oestrogen dominance may or may not involve low progesterone. You will see how this is possible when we talk about the liver. For now, simply know that the typical symptoms of *low progesterone* include:

- premenstrual migraine

- PMS-like symptoms (as outlined below under typical symptoms of oestrogen dominance)
- irregular or excessively heavy periods
- anxiety and nervousness
- feeling like you can't get your breath past your heart.

The typical symptoms of *oestrogen dominance* (which usually also involves low progesterone, but not always) include:

- irregular periods or excessive vaginal bleeding
- bloating/fluid retention
- breast swelling and/or tenderness
- decreased libido
- mood swings, most often irritability, easy to anger, and/or depression
- weight gain, especially around the abdomen and hips
- cold hands and feet
- headaches, particularly premenstrually
- tendency to yellow-tinged skin.

And all of these symptoms can lead you to feel lousy and like the lights have gone out in your eyes. On top of the internal impacts, the toll hormonal imbalances can take on your skin can have a significant ripple effect in a woman's life. When your skin is not great, whatever your age, it can be the source of immense frustration and stress. For countless women, balancing their sex hormones is key to a beautiful complexion.

The various forms of oestrogen dominance described above are the most common ones I see in menstruating women. The significant excess of oestrogen being made within the female body, combined with increased oestrogen in our environment (in food and chemicals, such as pesticides), appear to be affecting our endocrine (hormonal) systems in life-changing ways. The impact of this flows to the outside of the body and may present to you as a range of beauty challenges, from congested or pimply skin to a lack of zest for life.

It is essential to discern whether a woman is suffering from symptoms of oestrogen dominance caused by excess oestrogen, or by significantly low progesterone levels. For the latter it would mean that adrenal and/or ovarian production of progesterone is poor. This person may have optimal oestrogen levels, yet they are challenged with their periods due to low progesterone levels. The hormones that signal ovulation to occur are made by the pituitary gland, making optimal progesterone production reliant on good communication between the pituitary and the ovaries.

Another extremely common scenario is one of oestrogen excess. This can be due to excessive environmental exposures, including to plastics and/ or pesticides, and the use of oral contraceptives or hormone replacement therapy. Another significant basis for oestrogen excess is oestrogen recycling as a result of poor oestrogen detoxification by the liver. The liver actually decides whether to excrete or recycle oestrogen, and since it prioritizes what it needs to detoxify to keep you well and because the body makes oestrogen itself, detoxifying oestrogen is not as high a priority as, for example, the detoxification of alcohol. Hence, one reason why there can be so much oestrogen being recycled. A woman can have this month's oestrogen circulating, as well as last month's, and even oestrogen from numerous previous months. Even the best progesterone producer cannot balance and keep up with so much oestrogen.

An additional oestrogen-dominant hormonal picture is a combination of both the descriptions above of poor progesterone production and recycled oestrogen. If we took better care of our liver, this would be far less common in the Western world. As I love to say, these things have become common, but they are not normal. Women are not supposed to get PMS. Your period is just supposed to arrive — no extreme mood swings, no pain, no skin outbreaks, no premenstrual migraines — just menstruation. There are more free articles about sex hormones at: www.drlibby. com/bioresources

The following is an article I wrote for Breast Cancer Awareness Month. The brief I was given was to write about what makes breasts healthy. Some of it repeats information I have included earlier, but I have left it here in totality to remind you of how vitally important these factors are — and because breast cancer is tragically the leading cancer killer among women between the ages of 20 and 59 in high-income countries, the same population affected by PMS.

Healthy Breasts

When it comes to breast health, there is so much we now understand that contributes to the creation and maintenance of healthy breast tissue. Empowering women to take charge of this incredibly important aspect of their health is vital to the future of all women, and education must begin at a young age. Part of the challenge is deciphering fact from fiction or fad, so let's explore what we know creates healthy breasts.

Hormones, Stress, and the Liver

Although the hormone oestrogen does some wonderful things for our health, too much of it or too much of a particular type of oestrogen has been linked to some breast cancers. What is important to explore, when it comes to our hormones, is why is oestrogen so much more of a problem now as opposed to a time in the not-so-distant past? Part of the explanation lies in the production of stress hormones, and part of the explanation lies with the excretion of oestrogen following liver detoxification of this substance.

When we are stressed, we make either, or both, of our two dominant stress hormones, namely adrenalin and cortisol. As a result, levels of another sex hormone called progesterone, which has been shown to be protective against breast cancer (except those that are progesterone receptor positive), fall through the floor as the body links progesterone to fertility. If the body believes that your life is in danger and that there is no more food left in the world, the last thing it wants for you is a pregnancy. And so begins part of the problem with oestrogen — it is dominant in comparison to progesterone. This situation may also arise from synthetic forms of oestrogen, such as from the oral contraceptive pill (OCP) or hormone replacement therapy (HRT).

The second scenario to consider involves the excretion pathway of oestrogen out of the body. Once a molecule of oestrogen has done its job for a specific time, it is transported to the liver where it has to be transformed so that it can be excreted. There are two phases to this detoxification process. Over the years, the workload of the liver in its second stage of this cleaning process can get clogged, just like traffic on a motorway. Where once substances flew through the liver at, metaphorically speaking, 100 kilometres per hour (62 miles per hour), they might now crawl through at 20 kilometres per hour (12 miles per hour). When this process becomes terribly overloaded from years of too much alcohol, caffeine, refined sugars, trans fats, or the by-products of bowel congestion (a tendency to constipation), the oestrogen will undergo its first stage of change, but there is no room on the phase two highway, so the oestrogen is released by the liver back into the blood stream. Your body is then faced with the new oestrogen it continues to make from your ovaries — if you are still menstruating — and your fat cells, as well as the recycled form. It is this recycled form of oestrogen that has been found to be up to 400 times higher in women with oestrogen-sensitive breast cancer.

Looking after your precious liver is one of the best steps you can take to ensure that your breast tissue remains healthy. Sadly, many women regularly over-consume alcohol, and it is this regular, over-consumption that has been undeniably linked to the development of cystic breast tissue and breast cancer. Women need to get real about how much they are drinking. Heart organizations around the world suggest that two standard drinks per day (equivalent of two 100 mL [100 mL is equal to 3.4 fluid ounces] glasses of wine) with two days off each week is acceptable. Cancer research suggests, however, that if you have a family history of breast cancer, there is no safe level of alcohol consumption. That is a massive statement. If alcohol is something you enjoy, don't drink it daily. Save it for special occasions. Sparkling water with fresh lemon or lime can be a great, refreshing alternative.

Caffeine — coffee in particular — has also been found to play a role in the creation of denser, cystic breast tissue. On the other hand, green tea has consistently been shown in numerous studies to be protective against many types of cancers, breast cancer included. Most people are astounded at the changes in their breasts when they take a break from coffee and alcohol. As a woman living in the same world as all of you, a world with plenty of alcohol and caffeine on offer, I challenge you to take a break from these substances no matter how much you love or depend on them. Do it for one week, one little week out of your very long life. Once you've done that, do it for two. Or, better still, omit them for one or two menstrual cycles, and notice how different your breasts feel.

Food and Movement

When it comes to the aspects of our diets that are essential for healthy breast tissue, vegetables and fruits head the list. All of the cruciferous vegetables (Brassica family) have potent anticancer properties. Broccoli, in particular, contains sulphoraphane, a compound that helps the body begin to eliminate carcinogenic substances from the body in as little as ten days after it is included in the diet on a daily basis. It also keeps oestrogen from binding to and stimulating the growth of breast cancer cells, a vital step in keeping breast tissue healthy. The great news, too, is that sulphoraphane survives cooking. Eat broccoli, ladies!

Eat fruits and vegetables that are rich in beta-carotene. On average, women with breast cancer tend to have lower levels of beta-carotene in their blood, although researchers cannot say whether this is a cause or a result of the disease. A small-scale study in Italy found that beta-carotene given with other, related carotene compounds increased the tumour-free period among women who had already had breast cancer. The safest and most effective way to maintain healthy levels of beta-carotene is to consume five or more servings of dark-green, yellow, or orange vegetables and citrus fruits daily. We must eat our vegetables every day. No excuses!

Make an effort to minimize your consumption of fried foods and charcoal-grilled meats. Also, there is significant evidence to suggest that reducing the consumption of animal foods and basing your diet mostly on plant-based foods is incredibly beneficial to breast health and the prevention of breast cancer.

A growing body of literature suggests that insulin resistance is now a contributing factor in numerous cancers. Insulin is a hormone that can behave like a growth factor. It encourages all cells to grow: fat cells, healthy normal cells, and cells that may be pre-cancerous or cancerous. The best way to limit insulin production in the body is to never base a meal purely on carbohydrates or rely on processed foods. The only carbs humans ate up until the very recent past were those from whole food sources such as berries, legumes, and root vegetables. The barrage of highly processed foods, rich in refined sugars, starches and artificial ingredients we are faced with today did not even exist! Limit your intake of these. People also tend to forget that most alcoholic drinks are packed with sugar.

Remember it is what you do every day that will have the most impact on your health, not what you do sometimes. It is not about going without; it is about getting real about what you, as a woman, already know to be true. You know better than anyone when you have too much of a particular substance in your diet ... whether it is alcohol, coffee, or sugar. Make the changes you know you need to make now. You will give your breasts a great chance of remaining healthy in the process.

Lastly, move your body. The benefits of regular

movement are well documented for many areas of our health, including a reduction in insulin levels and body fat, both of which, in excess, have been linked to unhealthy breast tissue.

Nutrients for Healthy Breasts

Most of us have heard about the importance of iodine for optimal thyroid function and the prevention of goitre. What we hear very little about is how vital iodine is to breast health. The breasts concentrate iodine as do the ovaries, and studies have shown that the ovaries in an iodine-deficient state can produce a form of oestrogen associated with breast cancer. This has been shown to be reversible once iodine levels are optimal again. Use a salt that contains iodine, add seaweeds to cooking, or take a supplement to make sure you are getting your iodine. Be aware that you can have too much iodine but most people today aren't getting enough.

Also impacting breast health is our dietary intake and ratio of essential fatty acids. These are predominantly found in oily fish, flaxseeds, walnuts and pecans, evening primrose oil, and borage oil. It can be difficult to eat enough of these vital fats on a daily basis, so a good supplement combining at least fish or flax with evening primrose oils can be a great addition to your daily diet. Start with two capsules in the morning and two at night or one to two tablespoons of the liquid oil.

Another mineral that is essential for healthy breast tissue is magnesium and, coupled with selenium, these nutrients have been shown to reduce the incidences of new breast cancers. Green, leafy vegetables are high in magnesium, while Brazil nuts are rich in selenium. Eat them daily, or take a supplement.

Vitamin C is one of the most important nutrients when it comes to so many aspects of our health. The list of wonderful activities vitamin C performs in the body is almost endless. It helps keep the immune system responding appropriately to stimuli, and hastens white blood cell response times.

Vitamin B6 has also been extensively researched when it comes to breast health. Eggs are a good source, as are bananas and avocados.

Herbs for Healthy Breasts

Two of my favourite herbs work on the adrenal glands. These are Rhodiola and the Ginseng family. Both herbs are considered to be adaptogens, which means they help the body adapt to stressors by fine-tuning the stress response. These herbs tend to have a calming effect on the nervous system, which in turn promotes appropriate sex and stress hormone production, rather than extremes.

Other herbs that have been shown to be useful in creating healthy breast tissue are those that promote liver detoxification and bile production from the gall bladder. Bile is essential for the appropriate excretion of any fat-soluble substances from the body, including cholesterol and oestrogen. Useful herbs include St Mary's thistle, globe artichoke, Bupleurum, and Schisandra.

Minimize Exposure To ...

The final thing you need to know about the creation and maintenance of healthy breast tissue involves what is best kept to a minimum. Minimizing *exposure to growth-factor-like substances, including insulin, may be an important aspect of maintaining healthy breast tissue. Dairy products naturally contain growth factors. Cow's milk, for example, is designed to grow a 40-kilogram (88-pound) baby calf into a 900-kilogram (almost 2000-pound) beast. The growth factors naturally present in milk and milk products drive this growth. Humans, however, aren't designed to grow at these rates. If milk must be consumed, sheep and goats are smaller animals so their milks tend to drive slower, smaller growth rates. Alternatively, nut milks contain no growth factors.*

There is also a growing and very concerning body of evidence that points at the importance of minimizing our exposure to plastics and pesticides. They disrupt our endocrine systems and can mimic oestrogen. Recent research out of the United States shows that a large percentage of eight-year-old girls have hit puberty, leading to longer oestrogen production over their lifetime. Furthermore, as women choose to have fewer pregnancies or none, this can also lead to relatively more time spent in oestrogen-dominant states. Researchers suggest that poor diet, lack of exercise, high body fat, and exposure to plastics are the likely culprits for the earlier onset of menstruation. We can make a really big difference to our health and our children's health by getting these lifestyle factors on track.

~~~~~~~~~~~~~~~~~~~~~~~~

There are numerous reproductive conditions that involve poor progesterone production or oestrogen dominance in some way, and both of these scenarios have different effects on how a woman feels, and functions, and whether she feels like she looks her best. Endometriosis and polycystic ovarian syndrome (PCOS) are two of these conditions.

Endometriosis

Endometriosis is a condition where the cells that were intended to line the uterus migrate elsewhere outside the uterine cavity and adhere. Common sites for adherence are around the fallopian tubes, ovaries, bladder, bowel, pouch of Douglas (the area between the uterus and the bowel), and peritoneum. These cells respond to the hormonal signals communicating with the lining of the uterus and, as with the endometrium (lining of the uterus), the outlying cells thicken and fill with blood. When menstruation occurs, the cells outside the uterus also bleed, and this can be intensely painful and debilitating. Nine out of 10 women with endometriosis also have irritable bowel syndrome (IBS), which can be even more unpredictable during menstruation. Some newer theories about what is behind the condition involve the immune system, and I have no doubt that as research teaches us more about the causes women with endometriosis will benefit significantly.

Physiological Aspects

On a physical level, endometriosis is a condition of significant oestrogen dominance. That is, there is too much oestrogen, particularly in the second half of the cycle, compared to progesterone. As you now understand, progesterone doesn't just play a role in fertility but it is also a powerful anti-anxiety agent, an antidepressant, and a diuretic. Think about what life is like with very little of a hormone that plays all of these vital roles. Not much fun!

To get these sex hormones balanced for someone with endometriosis, the focus needs to be on both the liver and the adrenals. The liver makes the decision whether we excrete oestrogen or recycle it, and when the liver is too busy dealing with the typical liver loaders, as you will learn in the Beautiful Detox chapter, it tends to recycle the oestrogen. This means that, even for a good progesterone producer, it can be very difficult to have balanced hormones.

To remind you of the adrenal road to oestrogen dominance, it looks like this. For the first half of the menstrual cycle, oestrogen is supposed to be dominant. The adrenal glands are the only place we make progesterone from at this stage, but they also produce our stress hormones, adrenalin and cortisol. No matter what the reason is for your churning out stress hormones, your body will read it as meaning that the world is unsafe or there is not enough food. So because your body links progesterone to fertility, it therefore thinks it is doing you a great big favour by shutting off the adrenal production of progesterone. Remarkably, this doesn't always mean that you will have trouble conceiving, such is the power of the drive for the perpetuation of the species!

Notice that there are two biochemical scenarios involved in endometriosis. Breaking the oestrogen dominance cycle is key, and the road to hormonal balance can be quite different for everyone.

The following is a list of tests that can be useful in providing more insight into endometriosis. They certainly don't all need to be done at once, and diagnosis is typically made from a laparoscopy. But a good place to start investigating is with the hormones at the top of the list. They are:

- salivary hormone profile, including E1, E2, and E3 (this looks at three different forms of oestrogen)

- 2 and 16 urinary oestrogen metabolites (oestrogens are metabolized in two ways: the first pathway [2-hydroxyestrone] is protective, while the second pathway [16α-hydroxyestrone] is more potent, and this test identifies which is the dominant pathway (2 or 16) for oestrogen metabolism — the ideal ratio between the 2:16 pathways is 2-to-1)

- adrenal hormone profile, including cortisol

- CA-125
- serum protein PP14
- 25-OH-D_3 and 1,25-OH-D_3 (these are two different forms of vitamin D; typically in endometriosis, the 1,25 levels are deficient while the 25-OH levels are in excess — biochemically, this conversion relies on a process called hydroxylation which can be compromised in women with endometriosis)
- iron studies, B_{12}, folate, and full blood count
- MTHFR
- coeliac profile.

Dietary and Lifestyle Change: There are a few key nutritional factors that are essential for women with endometriosis: an anti-inflammatory way of eating that includes a high-plant diet and anti-inflammatory fats. Zero refined sugar is also key, and this can be a big challenge for women with endometriosis, as I have observed many who seem to have replaced self-love with sugar. I have personally witnessed almost miraculous improvements and, in some cases, complete resolution in women's endometriosis pain with dietary change, sometimes coupled with herbal support for the liver and adrenals. In some cases, women choose to have surgery first and then follow up with lifestyle changes, while for others, nothing improves until the emotional landscape has been explored. When you get it right, the body really lets you know.

Emotional Aspects

From an emotional perspective — and this is hard to write, but it comes from a place of love and deeply wanting to help — women with endometriosis may, on some level, blame others, usually their parents or partner for what happens to them. I find that one of their big life lessons is to truly learn to live from the space that life doesn't happen *to* them, but that life happens *for* them. No one else is responsible for them or for situations they find themselves in. Only they are. It is no one's fault. It can actually be quite difficult for women with endometriosis to see this aspect of themselves, but once they do I have seen the symptoms of the condition go and not come back, and I don't say that lightly. And I believe that happens because the insight the condition offered has fostered emotional growth that may not have been possible without it. That is why, when I describe clients who have had cancer and are now cancer-free, I call them cancer "thrivers", not cancer "survivors". Rock stars, actually.

If the frustration element above resonates, if you notice frustration is a common emotion for you, I offer you this: all emotions serve you. Those you may think of as "negative" emotions are merely calls to action. For example, if you feel frustrated, it may mean that you believe things could be better and they are not. This is a call to action telling you that there is something you could do now to make this better. This negative emotion is actually a gift if you use it effectively.

And if you recognize that you feel insecure regularly, I offer you this, via Steve Furtick, with much love: "If you struggle with insecurity, it may be because you are comparing your behind-the-scenes with everyone else's highlight reel." Really think about that.

Please don't get me wrong. What I'm sharing here is not suggesting you blame yourself for your illness. As Dr Christiane Northrup so beautifully says, "We are responsible TO our illness, not FOR our illness." Perhaps your illness has absolutely nothing to do with events in your life. To paraphrase Lissa Rankin, maybe you were just born with some lousy genes or you once lived next to a toxic waste dump or suffered from a tragic accident. I am not suggesting that your illness is your fault — not in the slightest. I am simply sharing with you an idea that I have seen assist others and that is that you explore your health challenges with a view to what they might teach you.

With regards to the emotional pattern that I find is common to endometriosis, it is important for you to know that if you still experience endometriosis after applying the nutritional, liver, and adrenal support strategies offered later in this book, it is not your fault! You aren't doing anything wrong. Live knowing that you are a beautiful soul, and trust that more insights will unveil themselves to you in time.

Polycystic Ovarian Syndrome

In polycystic ovarian syndrome (PCOS), the eggs in the ovaries ripen on the surface of the ovary but are not released. They harden and form cysts, hence the name of the condition. As you now understand, to obtain the optimal progesterone levels crucial for calm, fat burning, and your best sparkle, ovulation is essential, since the majority of your monthly progesterone is made by the corpus luteum.

Other hormones are also involved in PCOS. The pituitary gland makes luteinizing hormone (LH) and follicle stimulating hormone (FSH). Just prior to day 14 of a typical cycle, both hormones increase, but in PCOS both of these hormones from the pituitary gland tend to flat-line. Testosterone, the dominant male sex hormone, as well as other androgens, also tend to be higher in women with PCOS.

The LH and FSH hormonal profile of an ideal menstrual cycle is illustrated in the figure below, while the profile of someone with PCOS is represented in the second figure.

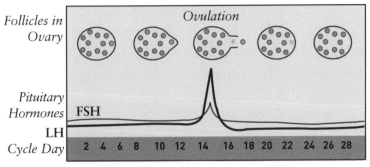

Ideal luteinizing hormone and follicle stimulating hormone peaks, generating ovulation: Both luteinizing hormone and follicle stimulating hormone peak to drive ovulation.

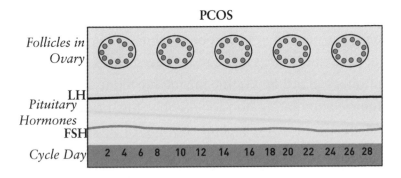

A typical PCOS luteinizing hormone and follicle stimulating hormone profile: Both luteinizing hormone and follicle stimulating hormone tend to flat-line in PCOS, with LH levels remaining consistently elevated.

When it comes to challenges with the reproductive system or hormones, I find exploring not only the biochemistry but also the subconscious beliefs and behaviours for each individual very useful and often the gateway to real change and health improvements. Nowhere is this clearer than in PCOS.

Physiological Aspects

From a hormonal perspective, in PCOS not only do the two pituitary hormones, LH and FSH, tend to flatline, but the other female sex hormones of progesterone and oestrogen also tend to be out of balance. Progesterone trends low while oestrogen tends to be high; however, there are also exceptions to this scenario where oestrogen is low as well (although, for almost all women with PCOS, oestrogen is still dominant over progesterone). The androgens, of which testosterone is one, tend to be on the high end of normal or elevated out of the normal range, sometimes dramatically so. And so it works like this: high androgen levels in the ovary inhibit FSH, which therefore hinders the development and maturation of eggs (in the ovary). At this stage in development, the "eggs" are called follicles. Dehydroepiandrosterone (DHEA), another steroid hormone, is found to be elevated in 50 per cent of women with PCOS. The elevated DHEA is believed to be due to stimulation by adrenocorticotropic hormone (ACTH), which is produced by the pituitary in response to stress. The excess DHEA then converts to androgens via adrenal metabolism and, in turn, contributes to the typical elevated androgen levels seen in PCOS. In working with women of any age with PCOS, we typically must first address cortisol production, as health and shine improvements unfold faster when what is at the heart of cortisol production is addressed. It is, however, important to note that not all women with PCOS have elevated cortisol. In fact, some have the adrenal fatigue picture described in the previous section. PCOS truly is a condition where the whole endocrine system can be involved; therefore, an individually tailored approach to getting the hormones balanced can be a game-changer.

The skin and adipose (fat) tissue add to the complex aetiology of PCOS. Women who develop hirsutism have the presence and activity of androgens in the skin, which tend to stimulate patterns of hair growth that might frustrate or sadden them, typically on the chin, the sides of the face, breasts, abdomen, and beyond the pubic area onto the thighs. Interestingly, 70 per cent of women in the United States with PCOS have hirsutism, while only 10 to 20 per cent of Japanese women do. Researchers believe that this may be due to both genetic and dietary factors, which reminds us yet again of another reason to eat a high-plant diet (like the Japanese).

With PCOS, the key to improvement usually

begins with focusing on stress hormone management. There are some beautiful herbs that might be highly beneficial in supporting this health picture. These include withania, licorice, rehmannia, and the nervine herbs passiflora, kava, and skullcap. Lavender can also be a lovely addition. Herbs are reviewed again in the Beautiful Solutions chapter.

Oestrogen dominance is well recognized as a metabolic feature for most women with PCOS, but just as important is addressing what is usually an elevated level of another hormone called prolactin. About 25 per cent of women with PCOS have hyperprolactinaemia (high blood levels of prolactin), which is due to the message the pituitary receives when oestrogen is elevated. High prolactin can then, in turn, contribute to elevated oestrogen. What a vicious cycle that one can be! Yet focus on now knowing where to start. In my experience, it can be tricky to catch prolactin elevated. It tends to follow cortisol somewhat, but, whereas cortisol will likely go high and remain elevated, prolactin seems to spike and fall away. A major tell-tale sign that prolactin keeps spiking is high breast sensitivity. This is particularly true in the lead-up to menstruation, but for women with PCOS, this breast sensitivity can last for weeks, rather than just a few days as it tends to with general PMS. There is a beautiful herb called chaste tree, also known as vitex, that can be highly beneficial in the regulation of prolactin (more about this in Beautiful Solutions).

If oestrogen is low in someone with PCOS, there are a number of theories about why this may be so, including genetics, poor transformation of cholesterol into oestrogen, and an altered hypothalamic-pituitary-adrenal (HPA) axis, which is the system that links those three glands via hormonal communication. Regardless of oestrogen levels, stress significantly impacts HPA axis function, and in some women with PCOS it is theorized that a possible outcome of overt or silent stress may be the formation of cysts on the ovary. There's also a blog post about PCOS at: www.drlibby.com/bioresources

I investigate all of these parameters with my clients, and I encourage anyone with symptoms that indicate PCOS to learn where they sit biochemically with all of these hormones. Therefore, the first step to getting your shine back to full sparkle may be some hormonal testing. The following is a list of tests that offer great insight into PCOS:

- salivary adrenal stress profile
- salivary female hormone panel, including testosterone, androgens, DHEA
- blood tests: FSH, LH, prolactin, E2, free androgen index (FAI) testosterone — free and total
- glucose tolerance test, fasting insulin, fasting

glucose (to determine if insulin resistance is present)

- thyroid blood panel: TSH, free T_4, free T_3, thyroid antibodies, spot urinary iodine
- blood lipid profile
- pelvic ultrasound.

Emotional Aspects

Exploring health conditions from an emotional and a metaphysical perspective often allows individuals to gain insight into any beliefs that may be behind their health condition. I find that it is often the combination of sorting out both the biochemistry and the beliefs that leads to beautiful results.

Think about this. There is nothing more feminine than our ovaries; men don't have them. With PCOS, however, it is as if the ovaries have gone deaf. The pituitary gland has been calling out to the ovaries in an attempt to alert them to release an egg — it is perhaps the most feminine process that goes on inside a woman. For the ovaries to no longer hear the call from the pituitary, there could be a silent, unconscious belief from somewhere in this person's world that they have to behave like a man in order to receive appreciation, connection, or love. Somewhere in their past, more masculine behaviour has been rewarded.

Women have shown they can match men in

every arena. But there are types of work that, even today, are still male-dominated. I have met countless women, working in what were previously more male-dominated roles, in particular, whose hormonal profiles have taken on a decidedly masculine appearance. These women are incredibly capable. The problem, however, lies in their — usually unconscious — beliefs about how they have to be in order to perform, achieve, and be loved. Most often, thinking or behaving "like a man" is in a woman's blind spot until we explore what that looks like. It is the mental approach to the work, not the work or job itself, which tends to be masculine.

Please don't get me wrong. I am not suggesting that all professional women have got, or will get, PCOS, nor am I suggesting that to be a woman and have a highly successful career means you have behaved like, or in the future will have to behave like, a man. What I simply want to point out is that your attitude, your perception of who you have to be, how you must behave, and what you have to achieve or do to get approval, is likely to be based on more masculine beliefs and behaviours. It may not have occurred to you that you even believe this, let alone that there is another way.

An Additional Note on Femininity

Our chemistry is ancient. What we ask of our bodies today is entirely different from what we asked of them even 50 years ago. On the one hand, it is truly remarkable what our bodies can do: work 16-hour days sitting at a desk, eat more processed rather than nutrient-dense food, breathe in more car fumes than ever before, all while we constantly think up solutions to challenges presented during the day, meet deadlines, juggle phone calls, crises, and complaints, and hopefully also celebrate a few things. And this is just the tip of the iceberg. On the other hand, we are so far removed from the way humans have lived for 149,950 years (if we've been on the planet for approximately 150,000 years) that I believe the human body is rebelling, and one of the most obvious areas is women's reproductive health, including fertility.

If this rings true for you, explore ways you can bring more feminine rituals into your life. What do you associate with femininity? For me, it is a light that shines in every woman. It is precious and oh so delicious. For me, masculinity represents direction, decisiveness, integrity, and presence. When you need to use masculine energy, for example at work, do it, but bring compassion into your heart and soften your gaze when you are there. No one will know this is what you have done. Don't look at the work on your desk and tense up. Instead, notice the work on your desk and take a long, slow breath that moves your belly when you inhale. Feel — and I mean really feel, really notice — how tension feels in your body. And then relax into it. Only you know you have done this. The feminine *feels*; and so many women have become so detached from their body that they are unaware of how they truly feel in their body. Your productivity and contribution will still be enormous, and most likely even more than what you found possible from a state of tension. Think about creating instead of producing. In emotional medicine, the ovaries are the seats of creativity. Just that shift in language is more feminine and can be helpful.

When you come home, as often as you can, be a complete girl! Light a candle and notice the fragrance. Dance around your house to music you love. Have a bubble bath. Giggle with the children or the tricks your dog wants to play, or at a comedy. Read a girly book if that appeals to you. Make a pot of herbal tea after dinner in a teapot you love, and turn it into an occasion. Notice the design of the pot and cup, the fragrance, and how you feel taking care of yourself. Masculinity (not men, but masculine energy) would never do this. But a man embracing his feminine would, just to point out the difference.

Please understand, this is not an anti-feminist concept, nor it is true for every woman with PCOS. I offer it as an observation of having worked with women for 15 years. Addressing the biochemistry of PCOS has enormous health benefits, including helping your shine. I simply wanted to highlight the incredible benefit I have also witnessed when women embrace their feminine essence in more areas of their lives. And feminine rituals are a beautiful place to start. I encourage all women with PCOS to explore what they perceive their fathers expected of them, or who they had to be in order to earn his love. And you will more than likely see that this is at the heart of why you do much of what you do. That may be OK, but it is no longer OK if this perception hurts your health. Enquire within about what is true for you. And then breathe, soften, and relax.

PUBERTY, PERCEPTIONS, AND OCPS

Some girls breeze through this time of transition without much change in their moods or their bodies, while for others an anxiety or even a darkness can set in. Oestrogen is the first female sex hormone to be made in any great quantity in a girl's body. As beautiful as oestrogen can be as a hormone, it can wreak havoc when it is present in substantial amounts for the first time ever in young female bodies that do not yet have sufficient progesterone being made to counterbalance its effects.

Prior to menstruation beginning, oestrogen production causes the breasts to bud and pubic hair to grow. It also begins to drive fat storage for all of the reasons outlined earlier. Some girls appear to be fleshier for a time just prior to menarche, indicating oestrogen is fulfilling its role.

Because progesterone is a powerful anti-anxiety agent and an antidepressant, if its production is slow to be initiated, a girl who was once bouncy, bright, full of energy, and interested in things, can become flat or anxious in her moods and distant in her relationships.

Oral Contraceptive Pill

If a girl's periods do begin and they are irregular and/or heavy and painful to the extent that she is unable to cope with school or life in general, she will often be encouraged to go on the oral contraceptive pill (OCP). It is important to understand two things here. One is the way in which OCPs work, and the second is the biochemical process that occurs at the onset of menstruation.

Physiological Aspects

First, the OCP is successful at preventing pregnancy because it shuts down the ovarian production of hormones, and ovulation cannot occur. The number of women of all ages I meet who have no idea how this powerful medication works astounds me. I am neither pro-pill nor anti-pill; I simply want people to make informed choices. I will say it again: the pill shuts down ovarian production of hormones, and the body relies entirely on the synthetic version of hormones being supplied by the tablet. Substances in patented medications, such as the pill, must be at least 10 per cent different from the form the body naturally makes. They are not identical to the form created by the body.

With the ovaries shut down and no progesterone production occurring from there, the adrenal production of progesterone becomes even more important, yet is unlikely to be optimal given what can be a stressful time for some girls. For starters, the onset of menstruation can increase a young girl's body fat for the first time. Never, never, *ever* comment on an adolescent girl's changing shape and size, or encourage her to eat less. That stresses her even more, as she may feel as though she is letting you down; it doesn't matter whether you are her parent, teacher, or friend. Explain that for a while hormones can change our shapes, and eating nutritious food and staying active are the most important things to do to stay healthy and keep glowing. All girls want to shine. Tell her not to worry about any changes she might notice, and demonstrate your love for her with your actions not just words. With less stress and the certainty of being loved, her progesterone is more likely to kick in, and her body shape and size will sort itself out. Some areas that can be useful to explore in this situation is an adolescent female's perception of academic pressure and her perception of what it may mean to a family member if she "fails" (which may mean not coming out on top of her class in some cases). Exploring what her "friends" are saying at school can also prove insightful.

Biochemical Aspects

The second issue that needs to be explored is the biochemistry associated with the onset of menstruation. This is the first time in a girl's life that her pituitary gland sends signals to her ovaries. For approximately the first five years, the chemical messengers released by the pituitary follow a road to the ovaries that looks like a goat track, meaning that it is a path that sometimes reaches a destination, in this case the ovaries, and sometimes winds up heading off into no-man's-land. In other words, sometimes the pituitary signals miss their mark. After about five years, this pathway, if it has been allowed to become established, behaves like a five-lane highway. The route is clear, straight, and unhindered.

What I see repeatedly, though, are girls who have

gone onto the pill to manage irregular or very heavy periods, rather than for contraception, shortly after menstruation begins. If sport is a big issue, or severe period pain is causing an adolescent girl to miss school, well-meaning adults, and/or health professionals in the girl's life may suggest that she go on the pill. But the pill simply masks the truth. If a girl stays on the pill long-term, the five-lane highway is never established. She will then come off the pill in adulthood, potentially wanting to have babies, but her pituitary has no history of communicating with her ovaries. It is a lot to ask our ovaries to suddenly wake up when we have suppressed their function for an extended period of time. It is wonderful if a teenager can be guided with nutritional medicine to resolve her challenging cycle. It would be wonderful if we could respond when our body first whispers to us that there is a challenge, rather than waiting for it to shout.

I cannot encourage you enough to get to the bottom of *why* the pain or the irregularity occurs in the first place. Before deciding whether or not the pill is the best choice, explore other options and seek ways to change the hormonal imbalance that may be present, or at least give the pituitary-ovary pathway time to become established.

Emotional Aspects and Holistic Approaches

So far as moods are concerned, what breaks my heart is seeing a young woman who has started menstruating, with heavy periods and some weight gain despite eating well, who disappears into her mind with her own private focus on sad thoughts, and an anxiety that often comes out with nervous-type behaviours, such as picking at her fingernails. This can be the first time ever that a girl experiences a tendency to depression or anxiety, and her family is often bereft and concerned at the change in their girl. The most common intervention in this situation is the prescription of the pill. But because the pill does not correct what is likely to be slow-starting or insufficient progesterone, the young woman's mood doesn't lift, despite her periods now being regulated by the pill. So she is encouraged by well-meaning adults to take an antidepressant. She is not even halfway through her teens, and she is on two of the world's most powerful medications.

There are times when conventional medicine is life-saving, and I am not suggesting it be avoided at all costs, especially not at the cost of precious human life. What I am encouraging, initially, is the balancing of oestrogen and progesterone through natural methods, with the support of an experienced health professional. Counselling at the same time may also be incredibly beneficial to assist with the new darker thoughts that may have arisen. My holistic approach means also discussing any fears the young woman may have about her perception of what it means to be an adult woman. It can be the first time she ever feels fleshy, puffy, or bloated, and, to a young mind influenced so heavily by popular magazines it is easy to understand why she can think she is fat when all she is, is oestrogen-dominant. As I said earlier, it is not physically possible to gain three kilos (six pounds) of fat in one day. It is most likely due to fluid and, given the diuretic action of progesterone, a deficiency of this vital hormone is one of the likely culprits of this young woman's fleshy feelings.

VITAMIN AND MINERAL DEFICIENCIES LINKED TO THE OCP

It is also incredibly important when it comes to health, inside and out, to be aware that the pill can deplete numerous vitamins and minerals in the body, as discussed below.

Vitamin A (retinol)

Various studies have shown disruption to vitamin A levels in the blood. Some show increases in retinol levels, which may simply mean less of the vitamin is stored in the liver. Other studies show a marked reduction in beta-carotene, the precursor to vitamin A. The implications are not yet clear for those on the pill. Eyesight changes can result from a deficiency in vitamin A, as this vitamin is needed for the normal, healthy functioning of the eyes. Increased susceptibility to infections, dry and scaly skin, lack of appetite and vigour, defective teeth and gums, heavy menstrual bleeding, cervical problems, and retarded growth are also linked to a deficiency. Vitamin A also acts as an important antioxidant and anti-cancer vitamin.

Vitamin B$_1$ (thiamin)

Although studies are inconclusive, there is a high probability that OCP takers are deficient in vitamin B$_1$. Signs and symptoms include fatigue, weakness, insomnia, vague aches and pains, weight loss, depression, irritability, lack of initiative, constipation, oversensitivity to noise, loss of appetite or sugar cravings, and circulatory problems.

Vitamin B$_2$ (riboflavin)

The body's requirements for vitamin B$_2$ are increased by use of the pill, which, if not addressed, can lead to deficiencies. The implications of this include gum and mouth infections, dizziness, depression, eye irritations, skin problems, and dandruff.

Vitamin B$_6$ (pyridoxine)

Depletion of this nutrient among women on the pill ranges from marginal to severe. Symptoms include nausea, low stress tolerance, lethargy, anxiety, depression, weakness, nervousness, emotional flare-ups, fatigue, insomnia, mild paranoia, skin eruptions, loss of muscular control, eye problems, and oedema (the excessive build-up of fluid, common in the feet and ankles). Vitamin B_6 is a nutrient that is critical in the conversion of tryptophan to serotonin, a brain compound (most of which is made in the gut) that significantly influences our happiness, calm and contentment, our pain response, eating patterns, moods, sleep patterns, psychological drive, and sexual desire. Vitamin B_6 is also needed for blood glucose management, the prevention of blood clots, and the maintenance of homocysteine at healthy levels (explained below).

Folic Acid

Research shows that levels of folic acid are significantly reduced on the pill. The most concerning and severe problem resulting from this deficiency arises when conception takes place while a woman is on the pill, or in the immediate period following, when the body is still recovering its folic acid stores. Since folic acid is required by the body to facilitate cell division, a process that begins immediately after conception, if this nutrient is deficient there is a much higher risk of abnormal synthesis of DNA and congenital abnormalities, including neural tube defects, spina bifida, deformed limbs, and mongolism. Deficiency can also lead to damage to the wall of the small intestine, anaemia, and elevated homocysteine levels, which have been associated with heart disease, various gynaecological conditions, and repeated miscarriage. Homocysteine can be maintained at healthy levels if folic acid and vitamins B_6 and B_{12} are in adequate supply.

Vitamin B_{12} (cobalamin)

Levels of vitamin B_{12} tend to be lower in pill users, and more commonly in those who also eat a vegetarian or vegan diet, while on the pill. The resulting effects include anaemia, a sore tongue, weight loss, depression, and elevated homocysteine levels.

Vitamin C (ascorbic acid)

I absolutely *love* vitamin C. All nutrients are essential (of course), but this one is super special for me, particularly when it comes to your shine. The pill increases the destruction of vitamin C. Levels can be reduced by up to 30 per cent, and this is made worse by smoking, stress, high pollution levels, infections, and some medications. A deficiency can result in bruising, bleeding gums, spider veins, heavy menstrual bleeding, eye problems, loss of appetite, muscular weakness, anaemia, fatigue, and a lowered immune response.

Vitamin C is also essential for the production of sex hormones, something your body will need to do more of itself if/when you no longer take the pill. A deficiency can make it far more difficult for your body to resume normal sex hormone production. Additionally, the lack of bioflavonoids that tends to occur when vitamin C is deficient (as they are usually found together) can exacerbate many of these symptoms.

Ironically, if vitamin C is taken in high doses (considered to be more than 2 grams per day), it can interfere with the effectiveness of the pill. This is because vitamin C increases the potency of the hormones, so when the dosage of vitamin C is reduced, your body can misinterpret this as a reduction in hormone levels, and ovulation may occur.

Vitamin E

There is an increased need for vitamin E as a result of oestrogen levels being higher when you are on the pill. Vitamin E actually helps to normalize oestrogen levels. The impact of insufficient vitamin E includes anaemia, muscle degeneration, subsequent low fertility, changes in the menstrual cycle, and hot flushes (flashes). Vitamin E is also necessary to help offset the greater risk of blood-clot formation and the possible carcinogenic effect of some forms of oestrogen. Selenium is critical for this anti-cancer role, as it needed for the body to be able to absorb vitamin E. Selenium levels are also decreased by the pill.

Calcium

Absorption is improved while on the pill. Although this may seem like a positive, it can further imbalance overall nutritional status.

Magnesium

Levels of magnesium are reduced in those taking the pill. Deficiency can cause a variety of premenstrual symptoms, lumpy breasts, muscle cramps, anxiety, sleeplessness, chocolate or sugar cravings, and cardiovascular problems.

Copper

While on the OCP, absorption of copper is increased, pushing the body's need for vitamin C even higher. Elevated copper disrupts the zinc-to-copper balance in the body, which can lead to symptoms such as insomnia, depression, migraine, and hair loss, as well as the possibility of high blood pressure and clotting tendencies.

Zinc

As you learnt in the Beautiful Nutrients chapter, zinc is another superstar nutrient when it comes to your shine. Levels of zinc are significantly lowered by the pill, which can lead to poor blood glucose management, sugar cravings, loss of appetite, poor resistance to infection, skin infections, lowered fertility, and a wide range of other problems. This mineral is critical for normal growth, cell division, tissue repair, and wound healing. If skin scars easily, I am always suspicious of a zinc deficiency.

As an aside, zinc is very important during pregnancy, as it is involved in over 200 enzyme systems in the body and is crucial for the healthy development of brain function and a competent immune system in a growing foetus; another reason to avoid conceiving while on, or soon after using the pill. In my experience, long-term pill-takers can find it difficult to rebuild their zinc status to adequate levels. This is certainly not the case for every woman, but I have had numerous clients take around three years to restore optimal zinc levels.

MENSTRUATION AND REST

Many women already know what I am about to share with you, and perhaps you have observed this in yourself: menstruation can be a time of soothing, stilling calm, a natural bliss. With some care and attention from you, this time can become your own natural, built-in zone to de-stress and regather your glow, if you feel it wandered out the door recently, or if you haven't been to bed before midnight for the past two weeks!

In our 24/7 lifestyles it is more important than ever to create islands of calm — time-out in which to release tension and simply be for a while. Just as we can't go without sleep for too long, your psyche cannot push on for too long without some quality downtime. The time you menstruate is the classic cyclic downtime due to the hormonal pattern and the energetics that exist at that time. One of the hormones involved in this cyclic downtime is called oxytocin, also known as the love hormone, as it engenders feelings of love, calm, and belonging. It is released at other times as well such as during sexual activity, childbirth, and breastfeeding, as well as when we touch, hug, or share a meal. Orgasm also causes oxytocin levels to rise from three to five times higher than baseline, creating feelings of closeness and tenderness after lovemaking. Oxytocin is also released at menstruation, as the uterus contracts at this time of the cycle, offering us a natural calm.

For so many women today, however, the lead-up to their period is a source of great despair, pain, misery, temper outbursts, and tears. Yet even with these states of upset (which I want so much for you to be relieved of ... please follow the advice later in the book, as you do not need to put up with menstrual cycle challenges!), if you were to pause you would notice that a calm state is available to you at this time.

In the West, we have an epidemic of exhaustion. We push and push and push, and don't allow ourselves enough downtime. There are few women in the Western world who would not benefit enormously from more rest. For women, menstruation is the natural time for this and, as a bonus during this time, an innate natural calm is on offer. Lifestyle changes may need to be made, however, to soak up the benefits of what your body is offering.

Slow down as you come into, and during, menstruation. Go to bed earlier. Apart from getting good-quality rest, there is evidence that the extra dream-time is good for easing PMS. Sleep is the all-round number one remedy, and it is free.

One of the strategies I suggest to women is to keep track of their menstrual period and reduce their commitments in the lead-up to and during that time, particularly on day one of bleeding. Even if you have to go to work, do your best to not push yourself too hard that day. If what I have just written makes you roll your eyes and exclaim on the inside that I clearly have no idea what your life is like, take a breath. There are very few women in the Western world who don't have 60 million things on their plate. But every minute of every day, you *choose* how to spend your time. Granted, it may not be possible every single month to give yourself the gift of some downtime during menstruation, but do everything in your power to make this happen. Your body's innate wisdom guides you to do this. Women need to allow themselves to be guided by their deep knowing more often. Even just doing this, I have seen women have far more regular, less challenging menstruation. For girls or women with PCOS who may not menstruate, I suggest you schedule your downtime for the first night of the dark moon. Science and history teach us that the ovaries are stimulated by light. Historically, before electric light, women tended to ovulate on the full moon and bleed on the dark moon. I encourage all women to notice the moon as often as they can. If you have to go outside at night, don't just take the rubbish out or tend to the dog or run to your car, look up at the night sky and notice the moon. I encourage you to draw her silver light into your ovaries and imagine them being lit up. This is a particularly important exercise if you don't menstruate regularly. While you do this, be sure to breathe from the diaphragm. Combined with attention to diet and herbs, this very feminine ritual can be incredibly beneficial to menstrual cycle calm and health, and therefore to your shine.

Scientific research supports the need for more quiet time in general. A day of absolute solitude was found to be the best antidote for what were shown to be "overtaxed, overstuffed brains" and the ideal way to attain optimal brain performance. Another researcher claimed that "everyone in the study was chronically stimulated, socially and physically, and that we are probably operating at a stimulation level higher than that for which our species evolved". This scientist's remedy was to spend more time alone. Two other scientists also found that attentive listening to silence helps the human brain focus, while what has been coined "conscious menstruation" by brilliant authors Jane Bennett and Alexandra Pope, some concepts from which were touched on above, has also been found to be a way to attain optimal brain performance.

Slowing down and becoming more conscious are crucial to our well-being. If we ignore our need to relax and avoid seeking solitude during menstruation, it may contribute to the development of some of the classic PMS symptoms such as disorientation, dreaminess, fogginess, feeling overwhelmed and irritable, as well as headaches and menstrual pain. However, if you can see your period as a time to turn down the volume, take a break, or perhaps just do less, the beauty and calm on offer will find you.

One of my clients, who insists on going to the gym seven days a week, decided to walk in Nature instead on the days of her period to see if that helped. It has, and she has now embraced this new ritual. Another lady got her closest friends together and asked them all to share their menstruation dates. They all plugged the dates into their phones and they make a point of getting in touch on the day their friends' periods are due to see if there is anything they can do to help out such as minding their children for a period of time that day. How gorgeous is that? Women are amazing.

Even if you lead a high-pressured life with barely a moment to yourself, with only a simple change in attitude you can start to get a taste of the natural calm on offer to you at the time of your period. The next time it is day one of your cycle, the first day of bleeding, take a moment before you race (hopefully not!) into your day, and notice how your body feels to you. Just acknowledge whatever you notice. Ask yourself what you would most love to do if you didn't have to work or worry about others that day. Then — with curiosity rather than despair, drama, or frustration — consider how you might give yourself 20 minutes of whatever that is on that day. When I have asked women this, the majority reply that they would love nothing better than simply curling up with a great book or a pile of magazines and not having to worry about anything or anyone. So ladies, please, examine your schedule and be ruthless about cutting out what is not essential on the first day of your period, even "fun" things like catching up with a friend for lunch. Notice how you might leak energy by getting caught up in drama, gossip, or having to listen to other people's problems. Do your best to excuse yourself from these situations as quickly as you can, for this is the one day you need to *receive*. Do your best to eat well on this day, too. At first, simply become aware of this pattern each month. The more aware of this cycle and this opportunity for calm you become, the more you will feel as though you can make little changes that will open this stage up for you, and the more effective you are also likely to be in your professional life. Renewal and rest are crucial to our health and our shine. You now need to allow it.

MENOPAUSE

At its simplest level, menopause is the cessation of ovarian production of hormones. But production continues from the adrenal glands and fat cells. However, as explained earlier, many women now make insufficient amounts of progesterone from their adrenals because of chronic stress. In my opinion, this is such a powerful factor in whether a woman breezes through menopause with few or no debilitating symptoms, or whether the heat and the sleeplessness become overwhelming. If you are approaching menopause, I cannot encourage you enough to ensure that your adrenal function is optimal. Apply the Restorative Foundation techniques described in the Beautiful Solutions chapter to help support the adrenal glands, and use breathing strategies and herbal support, combined with lifestyle changes where possible.

If you are postmenopausal, address adrenal and liver health, with the strategies discussed in the Beautiful Solutions chapter. Heat from the body can certainly be due to low oestrogen levels, low progesterone levels, and/or liver congestion. If I meet a client who has tried all sorts of natural oestrogen therapies and used herbs that have an oestrogenic action, such as black cohosh, and they are still overwhelmingly hot and suffering debilitating hot flushes, I will suggest treatments that support their liver.

Remember that in traditional circles, menopause is a time when wisdom begins to flow constantly. Trust what you already know inside of you when it comes to your health. You innately know better than anyone else what is best for you. Seek guidance from health professionals, but apply only what makes sense to you, and live knowing you are a shining light for the generations born after you.

A TIME TO SHINE

Menstruation and menopause are feminine and very natural processes. They offer incredible insight into a woman's general health as well as a window into her inner world of subconscious thoughts and beliefs. These thoughts and beliefs drive so much of what we do and how we feel. They can be a barometer guiding you to remember what you were born knowing: that you are the embodiment of loveliness.

Our behaviour is the outermost expression of our beliefs, and sometimes our hormonal balance as well as our shine can be returned to their naturally glowing state when we change what we believe we have to do to be loved. You don't have to "do" anything. Just be. For you are love. And you are light. It is time to allow your beautiful light to shine.

The most beautiful people we have known are those who have known defeat, known suffering, known struggle, known loss, and have found their way out of the depths. These persons have an appreciation, a sensitivity, and an understanding of life that fills them with compassion, gentleness, and a deep loving concern. Beautiful people do not just happen.

Elisabeth Kubler-Ross

Chapter 4
Part 3
Beautiful Thyroid Hormones:
how they impact your shine

When it comes to our sparkle, the thyroid gland is another part of the endocrine system that both contributes to, and is affected by, our environment and our perceptions. And again the pituitary gland, in this case influenced by the hypothalamus, controls thyroid function. Understanding where any dysfunction may have come from and the mechanisms involved are crucial to improving your health, your body size, and how you look and feel on a daily basis. Skin tends to be very dry, for example, if the thyroid is not working optimally, and it can also lead to hair thinning, not to mention a deep fatigue and a cold in your bones.

The thyroid is a little butterfly-shaped gland that sits in your throat area. It makes hormones that play an enormous role in your metabolic rate as well as temperature regulation and energy (that is, not feeling fatigued). Every day of my working life, I meet people who exhibit virtually every symptom of an under-active thyroid, yet their blood test results demonstrate that everything is in the "normal" range. More on "normal" ranges later.

THE THYROID HORMONES

The production of thyroid hormones involves a cascade of signals, and glands other than the thyroid are also involved. This means that if you have a problem with thyroid hormone levels, or with debilitating symptoms indicating that something is awry with your thyroid function, then it is essential to get to the heart of the matter so treatment can be appropriately targeted.

The thyroid function cascade begins with the hypothalamus, a gland that makes a hormone that sends a signal to the pituitary gland, the tiny gland that sits at the base of your brain, which we have already seen produces hormones involved in menstruation. The pituitary in turn makes a hormone called thyroid stimulating hormone (TSH) that signals the thyroid to make one if its hormones, known simply as T_4 (thyroxine). T_4 is found in the blood in two forms, namely T_4 and free T_4 (fT_4). They are the same hormone, except one is free to enter tissues and the other is bound up and unable to enter tissues, which is where the work needs to be done. However, T_4 and fT_4 are inactive hormones, and must be converted into T_3 and then the active thyroid hormone called fT_3 (free triiodothyronine). It is fT_3 that drives your metabolic rate and capacity to burn body fat. The flowchart below illustrates the hormonal cascade.

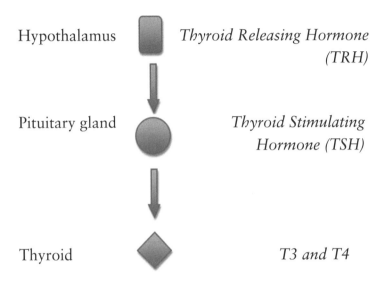

Hypothalamus	*Thyroid Releasing Hormone (TRH)*
Pituitary gland	*Thyroid Stimulating Hormone (TSH)*
Thyroid	*T3 and T4*

The thyroid hormone cascade: Signalling begins with the hypothalamus, followed by the pituitary, which then in turn signals the thyroid gland to make its hormones.

Here is a summary of various forms of thyroid hormones and their functions;

- TSH — reflects the blood level of thyroid stimulating hormone.

- Total T_4 — reflects the total amount of T_4 present in the blood; that is, the bound (unavailable) T_4 and the Free T_4. Note that high levels of synthetic oestrogens or oestrogen dominance can increase the amount of the protein that binds T_4. This may produce misleading elevated Total T_4 values, which can look like hyperthyroidism when it is not.

- Total T_3 — reflects the total amount of T_3 present in the blood; that is, the bound (unavailable) T_3 as well as the Free T_3. Oestrogen dominance creates the same effect as mentioned in relationship to T_4.
  Free T_4 — reflects the biologically active (free) form of T_4. This T_4 can be converted to T_3 or RT_3. This value is relatively stable and does not appear to be influenced by oestrogen dominance.

- Free T_3 — reflects the biologically active (free) form of T_3 that can generate production of energy (in the form of ATP). This value is relatively stable and does not appear to be influenced by oestrogen dominance.

- RT_3 — reflects the level of Reverse T_3. This can be measured; however, the approximate value can be estimated from knowing T_4 and T_3 values since T_4 will become either T_3 or RT_3. For example, if the T_4 is elevated and the T_3 is low, we know that RT_3 (what the rest of the T_4 becomes) will be relatively elevated, which is not what you want.

There are a number of nutrients essential to the production of optimal levels of thyroid hormones. Iodine and selenium are both vital minerals to this process of conversion that literally lights up your metabolic rate. Many people today get very little iodine and selenium in their diets as the majority of soils in the Western world do not contain these trace minerals, and if the nutrients are not in the soil they cannot be in the food that is grown in them.

The thyroid gland can become over-active, known as *hyperthyroidism*, or under-active, known as *hypothyroidism*, and it is the latter scenario that can lead to weight gain that can be difficult to shift until this issue is addressed. Both poles of dysfunction, however, can impact on your shine.

Some people swing between an under-active and an over-active situation. The thyroid gland is also susceptible to autoimmune diseases, meaning your immune system, which is supposed to defend you from infection, starts to see the thyroid gland as a foreign particle, like a germ, and attacks it, leading to a change in its function. This can lead to either the over-active picture (with autoimmune involvement this is known as Graves' disease) or an under-active picture (known as Hashimoto's thyroiditis with autoimmune involvement). Infection, poor liver function, iodine, selenium, and iron deficiencies, as well as oestrogen dominance and high or low cortisol levels, are all major factors that can initiate thyroid dysfunction. If you suspect your thyroid is not working optimally, re-read the list just outlined and think about what you have already learnt from the earlier sections about stress hormones and sex hormones and if they may be impacting on the optimal function of your thyroid. It is important to work out the path that leads someone to altered thyroid function, for behind the "why" lies most of the answer — the road into dysfunction is also the road we need to take out. If this doesn't make sense yet, it will very soon!

HYPOTHYROIDISM: UNDER-ACTIVE THYROID GLAND FUNCTION

One of the first things that springs to mind with under-active thyroid people, is that they almost always tell me that coffee makes them happy and that the first 20 minutes or so after they have had a coffee, is the only time they feel what they call "normal". They feel like they can function. They will also usually tell me that chocolate helps them, and, if they feel this way, it is potentially not just the caffeine content of the chocolate but maybe also the dopamine-enhancing actions of this food. Dopamine is a neurotransmitter that when in low supply can be involved in depression, while excessive amounts can drive addictive behaviours. For someone with poor thyroid function, chocolate may give them a little lift. Please don't assume, though, that if you love chocolate, you have a thyroid issue — many people simply love chocolate.

The classic symptoms of hypothyroidism are:

- gradual weight increase over months for no apparent reason, or weight that won't budge no matter what you do
- often feeling cold, sometimes cold in your bones and like you can't get warm
- tendency to constipation
- tendency to depressed mood, forgetfulness, and a sense of being easily confused
- hair loss or hair drier than previously
- dry, brittle nails
- menstrual problems
- difficulty conceiving
- beyond tired, you are fatigued
- headaches.

If a woman's thyroid gland is under-active, she is more likely to feel deeply fatigued and depressed in her mood, rather than racy and anxious. However, I have met countless women who, from a mood and behaviour perspective, appear to bounce between these two extremes, so I feel it is important to explore both the under- and the over-active thyroid health pictures. And given that the thyroid is controlled by the pituitary, when the whole endocrine system is not able to work optimally due to what might be a poor-quality diet, lack of restorative sleep, worry, and/or a perception of pressure, the thyroid is a likely target for dysfunction.

Let's explore the roads to an under-active thyroid and where to begin to support your thyroid health.

Infection and Poor Liver Detoxification

A history, at any stage in life, of glandular fever (Epstein-Barr virus, also known as mononucleosis) can be a common road to hypothyroidism. Another route is liver overload, or a congested liver as I sometimes refer to it. Treatment of both of these roads involves taking excellent care of the liver, and I encourage you to apply my liver-loving strategies! Additionally, astragalus is an excellent herb to use for a chronic infection background if an herbalist agrees this will meet your needs.

Mineral Deficiencies

Since hypothyroidism can be influenced by deficiencies in selenium, iodine, and iron, choose foods that are rich in these minerals. Eat Brazil nuts daily for selenium, and use Celtic sea salt with iodine and/or cook with seaweeds, such as kombu, for iodine. To review, good food sources of iron include beef, lamb, eggs, mussels, sardines, lentils, green leafy vegetables, and dates. There is a small amount of iron in many foods, so eating a varied diet is important. And remember that absorption is enhanced by vitamin C. If you do not eat animal foods, do not assume you are iron-deficient. For some vegetarians, their body utilizes the iron from vegetable sources very efficiently, but it is worth testing.

The other option is to take a supplement that covers these nutrients. There are some excellent thyroid support capsules on the market, and you could consult with a health professional if you are interested in trying that route. Regarding iron, it can be good to have a test before you supplement, as overloading on iron is not good. A test can be done for both iron and your iron storage (ferritin) levels. If you are deficient, it can be a challenging and very slow process to get your iron levels up without supplementation. So it is good to know your blood levels of this mineral. Many iron supplements are constipating, but most people find this doesn't happen with liquid iron supplements.

Here's more on iodine from a magazine article I wrote just so you know how important this is ...

Iodine

Iodine is a trace mineral so essential to our health that our body begins to shut down without it. Our thyroid gland loves iodine, and it cannot make thyroid hormones without it. Symptoms of an underactive thyroid include a deep tiredness, a sluggish, heavy feeling, dry skin or hair, feelings of cold, a ten-

dency to be constipated, puffy eyes, and a propensity to a depressed mood. Increasing dietary iodine intake can make a big difference, if iodine is an issue for you.

Thyroid hormones essentially determine our metabolic rate as adults and our growth as children. Iodine is also essential to the IQ of the developing brain in utero and, sadly, studies are now showing that some children in the Western world are suffering from such low iodine levels that their IQ is detrimentally affected.

Why is this so?

Soil is a poor source of iodine, and if a nutrient is not in the soil it cannot be in our food. Where once foods made from whole grains, for example, were good sources in areas where the soil contained iodine in the first place, the depletion of the mineral content of our soils means this is no longer the case. New Zealand, for example, has volcanic soil, which has never contained any iodine. While the soil may not be a good source of iodine, the sea is somewhat better.

Food sources of iodine include all of the seaweeds, which you can add to soups, stews, casseroles, and salads to give them a subtle salty flavour, while imparting their nutritional value. A form of seaweed commonly eaten is nori, used frequently in sushi. Seafood contains small amounts of iodine, but even eating seafood every day will not provide you with adequate amounts of iodine.

Salt was first iodized in 1924; however, it tended to go out of fashion with the advent of rock salts and Celtic sea salt. Although Celtic sea salt offers the additional benefits of a broad range of trace minerals, some brands lack iodine — unless it has been fortified. Himalayan pink salt tends to contain a great range of minerals, including iodine. The only concern with conventional iodized salts is that most brands contain anticaking agents that are not ideal for human health. Bottom line? Check your salt to make sure it contains iodine.

Iodine is a difficult mineral to test for. Accurate tests require you to collect 24 hours of urine and, remarkably, not all countries offer this testing.

Adult females require 120 micrograms (µg), males 150 µg, of iodine per day to prevent deficiency. It is far more beneficial, however, to individualize doses. Often higher doses are initially necessary to treat a deficient state, and this can easily be done with one to three drops of a good-quality liquid iodine solution per day, available from some health food shops or through a compounding pharmacist. It is best to be guided by a health professional to meet your individual needs.

~~~~~~~~~~~~~~~~

Oestrogen Dominance

Too much oestrogen can suppress thyroid function, while optimal progesterone levels support its function. Apply the strategies for dealing with oestrogen dominance if you suspect that this is the basis for your challenge with your thyroid gland. For example, if you have had challenging periods for a few years, you may have been oestrogen-dominant for that time, and this can lead the thyroid to not work optimally. If your thyroid dysfunction is due to oestrogen dominance, no amount of iodine or selenium will resolve it; only sorting out the oestrogen dominance will — road in is road out.

Elevated Cortisol Brought on by Stress

Elevated cortisol as a result of stress decreases the levels of the active, fat-burning thyroid hormone T_3, which slows your metabolism. Added to this, high levels of cortisol urge your body to break down muscle to provide glucose for your brain, and reducing your muscle slows your metabolic rate as well. In the absence of stress, a healthy body converts T_4 into T_3, but with elevated cortisol levels the conversion of T_4 to T_3 decreases.

Poor conversion of T_4 to active T_3 also occurs if you restrict your food intake. Your body assumes that you must be starving, and therefore it must slow down the metabolic rate to preserve those precious fat stores. It may be frustrating, but your body's primary goal is always survival.

Elevated cortisol can also inhibit the release of TSH from the pituitary and, with less TSH, the body usually produces less T_4. Apply the strategies to support the adrenal glands if this scenario rings true for you. Poor thyroid function can also lead to elevated cholesterol and, once thyroid function has been treated, the cholesterol returns to normal.

Low Cortisol Brought on by Stress

As you now understand from the Not-So-Beautiful Stress Hormones chapter, cortisol levels can also plummet, usually after prolonged stress. It is as if the adrenals crash. When this happens, the information the thyroid receives can also drive it to dysregulation and, for some, supporting the adrenals using herbs and nutrients, as well embracing a more calming way of life, can be the best "medicine" for the thyroid. In my practice I have often found women's thyroids respond better to thyroid treatment when the adrenals are supported at the same time.

Thyroid Medications

Typically today, if someone has been diagnosed with an under-active thyroid, they are prescribed thyroxine (T_4). Some people feel brilliant on this medication and all of their hypothyroid symptoms disappear, including what is likely to have been unexplained weight gain. If this has not happened for you despite taking this medication, try a different approach. After years of taking thyroxine, it will not suddenly start to work if it hasn't yet. Same goes if the fatigue hasn't lifted. In your journey to feel like your spark is ignited, you may need a different or an additional support.

There are numerous brands of thyroxine on the market. If you want to stick with conventional medicine, tell your general practitioner if you feel lousy on your current medication and communicate that you would like to try a different drug. I had hundreds of clients who were happily taking one form of thyroxine, and, when the thyroid medication that is subsidised was changed to a different brand, all of their symptoms returned. Explore this even if your blood levels of TSH, fT_4, and fT_3 are "normal", but you still have symptoms.

In my opinion, an excellent option to try when it comes to hypothyroidism is whole thyroid extract (WTE). This is taken instead of any synthetic medication and, unlike the synthetics providing only one of the thyroid hormones, WTE provides all of the thyroid hormones. If you are interested in exploring this, it is essential to work closely with your doctor during a transition in medications. Whole thyroid extract is made by a compounding pharmacist.

If you have not been diagnosed with a thyroid illness, but you exhibit numerous symptoms, do not rely solely on your blood test results to determine if your thyroid is under-active. Work with a health professional who will treat the symptoms, not the blood, and who will monitor both your symptoms and the blood work as you explore treatments. I learnt this in a powerful way with a client whose story melts my heart.

Patricia's Story — Thyroid Antibodies

The importance of testing thyroid antibodies is best demonstrated with this story. A precious lady arrived at my practice asking for assistance with her health. When I asked how I could help, she burst into tears and said she had known that she had an under-active thyroid for about 30 years. Patricia's blood tests always come back within the normal range, and no one would treat her. She had gained over 100 kilos (220 pounds) over the 30 years, and it all began when her dear mother passed away. Patricia said she had eaten poorly for about three to four months after her mother's death, and put on weight, but her grief gradually eased and, as it did, she started to eat better again, as she always had. But nothing changed. Her size kept increasing. So then she didn't just eat well, she signed up for a gym membership and she started to eat even better. When I saw her, Patricia was unable to exercise due to knee pain from carrying so much weight (her description, and she thought she was "about 180 kilograms" [400 pounds]), but she still ate in a way that did not warrant her size.

Of course Patricia had a huge amount of unresolved grief, to which, she said, doctors, with the best of intentions, kept offering her antidepressants. She always declined because she felt it was her thyroid. Yes, there had been times when she hadn't eaten very well. But she also had plenty of months and years of making extraordinary efforts for no reward.

Given that Patricia ticked every box when it came to symptoms of an under-active thyroid, I decided to request fresh blood tests and include thyroid antibodies, specifically anti-thyroid peroxidase and anti-thyroglobulin. Having been taught at university that it

*was highly unlikely for thyroid antibodies to be ele-
vated and an issue if thyroid hormone levels were in
the normal range, I could understand why Patricia's
auto-antibodies had not been tested — but from a
symptoms perspective, I could not.*

*To cut a very long story short, despite her lat-
est thyroid hormones levels being in the "normal"
range, but skewed one way (discussed below), Patricia's antibodies were the highest I have ever seen. To
put this in context, the "normal" range for both of
these antibody tests in this national laboratory is less
than 50. Patricia's anti-thyroid peroxidase and anti-
thyroglobulin were both greater than 6500 — off the
scale and through the roof. When I telephoned to tell
her, she was at first thrilled that all along there had
been a reason for how lousy she had felt. She told me
later that anger then surfaced for a life she felt she'd
missed out on because this was not picked up on. She
had remained very shy, which she blamed on her size,
and on reflection was very sad that she had not met
a partner with whom to share her life. She decided
to seek out the most natural approach she could for
her very under-active thyroid, and, after considerable
weight fell off her over the first three months, she
booked her first overseas holiday.*

There is always a why to how you feel. You just
have to find it.

HYPERTHYROIDISM:
OVER-ACTIVE THYROID GLAND FUNCTION

Common signs and symptoms of an over-active thyroid include:

- heart palpitations

- heat intolerance or easily over-heating (this can also indicate liver congestion)

- nervousness

- insomnia

- breathlessness

- increased bowel movements

- light or absent menstrual periods

- fatigue, but more wired than tired

- fast heart rate

- trembling hands

- weight loss (although not always, as appetite increases with hyperthyroidism and some people eat enough to cover the increase in metabolism)

- muscle weakness

- warm, moist skin

- hair loss

- staring gaze

- bulging eyes.

Thyroid hormones have a direct effect on most organs, including the heart, which beats faster and harder under the influence of elevated thyroid hormones. Essentially, all cells in the body will respond to increases in thyroid hormone levels with an increase in the rate at which they conduct their business.

When it comes to an over-active thyroid, whether there is autoimmune involvement (Graves' disease) or not, a frantic pace of life has been involved with every single case I have ever worked with. In my experience, stress, specifically the pace of life and what each woman has demanded of her body, is the major factor in the development of hyperthyroidism. More than any other group, they have sacrificed sleep and juggled more in their lives to date than most people could juggle in a lifetime. As I like to say to one of my favourite rushing friends, "it is as if you run a small country" with all that she handles. And there is usually a part of them that actually quite enjoys life this way. They are incredibly capable. They are often at a bit of a loss why their body has gone and done this; namely, presented with elevated anti-thyroid antibodies along with elevated thyroid hormone function tests. Yet their body has sent them a powerful message: the way in which they are living is not serving their health, or perhaps even their destiny, and what life has in store for them. I believe that your body does its best to wake you up to pay attention to what *really* needs your attention, every day. I have seen some over-active thyroid conditions return to normal with this acknowledgement and the subsequent lifestyle change that must go with it.

The women I have worked with who have successfully returned their thyroid function to normal from being over-active, and had a complete remission of their symptoms, have literally changed their life. Initially, they usually go on medication prescribed by their doctor, but, while on medication, make lifestyle changes with a view to using medication short term if they can. They usually change their jobs, and if that is not possible they completely change their approach and attitude to that work and their life. My observation is that they are usually very playful women who love a good laugh; incorporating this element of their personality into their everyday life, including at work, helps their health and their shine. This has been incredibly inspiring to witness in my clients. In *You Can Heal Your Life,* Louise Hay suggests that in hyperthyroidism there can be a feeling of "rage at being left out", and she encourages people to affirm: "I am the centre of my life, and I approve of myself and all that I see." Explore this if it resonates for you; but if it doesn't, simply move on.

It is virtually impossible to slow down and approach life from a calm, centred space when your body is getting the message that it needs to speed everything up.

It can be very difficult to take part in a meditation class when your heart feels like it is about to jump out of your chest. So the physical aspect of this condition most certainly needs to be sorted out. However, I want to encourage you to also get to the real reason of why you may have run your life at such an intense pace in the first place, a concept I explore in *Rushing Woman's Syndrome*.

BLOOD TESTS AND "NORMAL" RANGES

The concept of a "normal" range is necessary, as cut-off points help indicate when something may be abnormal. I have great concerns, however, when we base the future of a person's health on blood tests alone.

According to Dr Karen Coates, an insightful and pioneering general practitioner and co-author of *Embracing The Warrior: An Essential Guide for Women*, the normal range for some blood tests is calculated periodically by each pathology laboratory to ensure that the reference range printed on the test results is "accurate". On the morning of this day, the first 100 blood samples received are tested for their (in this case) TSH levels in order to determine the reference range. Or it might be iron levels, for example. But! Why do people usually have blood tests? Because they are feeling particularly spritely that day? No — most often the precise opposite is true! Yet it seems we base our "normal" ranges on these figures. Furthermore, it is also important to understand how the "average" amount of a particular nutrient or hormone is calculated. Mathematically, the top reference point is calculated to be "two standard deviations" above the average, while the bottom figure is "two standard deviations" below the average. The arbitrary rules of this method dictate that 95 per cent of the 100 blood samples taken must fall into the "normal" range. The statistical definition of standard deviations insists that only four or five results may fall outside of this reference range, two or three samples below and two or three above.

I want to make two points. First, the reference ranges for some blood parameters are getting broader. The normal range for TSH when I wrote the first draft of my book *Accidentally Overweight* was 0.4 to 4.0. By the time the book went to publication, four months later, the normal range had been expanded to 0.3 to 5.0. As mentioned later, people at either end of this blood range will look and feel completely different, and they will more than likely exhibit thyroid symptoms. If they are symptom-free, no problem, their body is not trying to draw their attention to the thyroid gland. However, my concern is this: if we base treatment on the blood work alone and leave people to live with their symptoms, with their result skewed to one end of the normal range, we are risking, not optimizing, their health. This brings me to my next point, which is that you can see from the start that this process is flawed, given it is undertaken on individuals who are potentially unwell. It is more challenging to create optimal health, prevent disease, and maximize quality of life for people when they are being guided with their blood tests to fall into a potentially unhealthy normal range.

YOUR BLOOD TESTS

I urge you to get copies of your own blood tests and look for results being skewed to one end of the normal range. Let me explain.

The normal range for TSH where I live is currently 0.4 to 4.0 (it switched back to this range). Although those numbers may seem small, someone with a TSH of 0.4 feels and looks completely different than someone with a TSH of 4.0. Additionally, if your results are not actually outside the normal range, you will usually be told, well-meaningly, that there is no problem with your thyroid. A common picture I see is a TSH of 2.5 or greater (made by the pituitary) screaming out to the thyroid gland to make T_4. Normal levels of T_4 are between approximately 10 and 20 units and, usually for someone with symptoms of hypothyroidism, their T_4 might be 11. This person feels exhausted in their bones, has trouble naturally using their bowels daily, has dry skin, very low motivation, a tendency to a depressed mood, brain fog, and their clothes are gradually getting tighter. They feel so far from their former selves, and I have met many women who wonder if they will ever get their gloss back. Their thyroid needs support, and when this is tailored to the individual, optimal health and a zest for life return.

In this case, I always start with iodine and selenium and sometimes iron, along with adrenal support, a grain-free diet, and a big chat about their beliefs and what their perception is of what life is like for them. If oestrogen has been dominant for some time, I also address that.

Sue's Story

A client came to see me for help with her debilitating fatigue and her inability to lose weight. She had been on thyroid medication for three years. Sue worked as a schoolteacher, was married, and had two teenage children. Her day consisted of dragging herself out of bed to go to work and, as soon as she came home in the afternoon, she had to go to bed and sleep, or she couldn't function the next day. She shared with me how grateful she was to her husband for his support, as he took care of all of the meals and the house, as well as helping the children in the evening. She had no quality of life and it also affected those around her. When I looked at her blood test results at diagnosis, this lady's TSH was 14.9 (normal range 0.4–4.0). After a year of working on getting the dose of medication right, her TSH had stabilized at either 7.8 or 7.9 and had sat there for two years. Sue had been told there was nothing more that could be done to both get her TSH lower and resolve her deep fatigue and the impact that was having on her life.

It was very clear to me that the first step for this lovely lady was a gluten-free diet, and I guided her to do this for a trial period of four weeks, after which time I suggested she have her thyroid hormone levels re-tested. After her TSH sitting at 7.8 or 7.9 for two years, with four weeks on a gluten-free diet her TSH was 4.8 and, even more importantly, she could now delay her bedtime until 9pm. Game-changing.

The next step was herbal medicine to support Sue's adrenals, as well as her thyroid, and four weeks later her TSH was 4.2, another wonderful drop and another improvement in how she felt, this time in how her clothes fit. This precious lady shared with me that she had not been able to lose weight for "at least 10 years" and now it felt effortless.

Like I said, there is always a reason — we just have to find what serves your inner and outer wellness!

And, finally, one last case study to demonstrate what thyroid support can do.

Karen's Story
A 24-year-old who had tried all sorts of things to solve her skin congestion reached out to me. She had read Rushing Woman's Syndrome and had learnt so much about how skin is simply a reflection of interior processes. Here is what Karen wrote:

My skin had been playing up. I assumed my skin wasn't good because of my diet so I really amped up green smoothies and greens in meals, etc. I also went *off fried foods and chocolate — and religiously took my fish oil and flax fibre with evening primrose oil and saw no change.*

So I bought some ThyAdren (selenium and iodine as well as herbs I'd read about in your book), as I felt I was probably lacking in iodine. I have noticed huge improvements to my energy levels but also my skin. The reason this is interesting to me is that technically I shouldn't have "low" thyroid function. My blood tests are normal, and I don't have any of the symptoms. I have no trouble losing weight. Made me wonder how many women like me with skin problems have suboptimal thyroid levels, particularly in New Zealand and Australia.

Quite often, the aspect of your outer appearance that frustrates you most is a great gift, asking you to eat, drink, think, or move differently, asking you to look beyond what you are currently doing to support your health. Now, not only has lovely Karen's skin returned to its flawless state, but now she also understands that this was made possible because her thyroid and adrenals are working optimally. And if those glands are left working suboptimally for long periods, they can have more significant health consequences down the track.

As touched upon earlier, Louise Hay, the brilliant metaphysical medicine pioneer, teaches that thyroid problems represent feelings and beliefs around humiliation and feeling like you never get to do what you want to do. (How many mothers, in particular, does that describe?!) Because I think addressing such issues are an essential part of an holistic approach, it is worth revisiting these ideas as a conclusion to this chapter. Louise Hay suggests someone with thyroid problems unconsciously asks: "When is it going to be my turn?" She proposes that you develop a new thought pattern of "I move beyond old limitations and now allow myself to express freely and creatively", and suggests people with hypothyroidism explore any feelings of hopelessness, a feeling of being stifled, or a sense of giving up. If it rings true for you, Louise suggests that you develop a new thought pattern of "I create a new life with new rules that totally support me." I encourage my clients who have a thyroid that needs support to know that every moment is, in fact, their turn, as one of the most transformational learnings in life is that life doesn't happen *to* you, life happens *for* you.

I include this information to offer you a whole picture of your thyroid health, one that covers the conventional function of hormones, glands, and blood tests, through to the nutritional supports that are essential, especially iodine and selenium, and yet also addresses the metaphysical. Somewhere among these three approaches lies your answer, not necessarily in just one or the other. I urge you to explore all three.

Promise me you'll always remember: you're braver than you believe, and stronger than you seem, and smarter than you think.

Christopher Robin (to Pooh)

Chapter 4
Part 4
Beautiful Pituitary Hormones:
their role in your glow

Part of what I always aim to do for people is get to the heart of their particular health matter, with the view to resolving or healing what they want to work on. I also always look for the bigger picture that this particular health and/or beauty challenge is offering. This usually involves exploring what is happening for an individual physically *and* emotionally.

There are numerous body systems intricately involved in our physical and emotional health, how we look, how we feel, and how we behave. And as you now understand, the nervous system and the endocrine system hold the key to so much about how we feel, how we see ourselves, and how others perceive us. The master control centre for our hormonal systems is the pituitary gland, a gland that is too often overlooked when exploring a woman's health, unless symptoms distinctively point to a problem in this area. Yet creating an environment inside the body that allows the pituitary gland to work optimally can be the key to a calm existence, one that allows great regulation of all the other endocrine glands, including the adrenals, the ovaries, and the thyroid, allowing you to sparkle inside and out.

WHAT DOES THE PITUITARY GLAND CONTROL?

The pituitary is a pea-sized gland located at the base of the skull between the optic nerves; its main task is to secrete hormones. The reason the pituitary is sometimes referred to as the "master gland" is because it controls hormone functions, such as our temperature, thyroid activity, growth during childhood, urine production, and ovulation. In effect, the gland functions as the thermostat that controls all the other glands that are responsible for hormone secretion. The gland is a critical part of our ability to respond to the environment. It is the link between our nervous and our endocrine systems. The chart below shows the location of the pituitary gland, housed in the brain at about level with the bridge of your nose, and the glands it affects.

The Pituitary and Its Target Glands

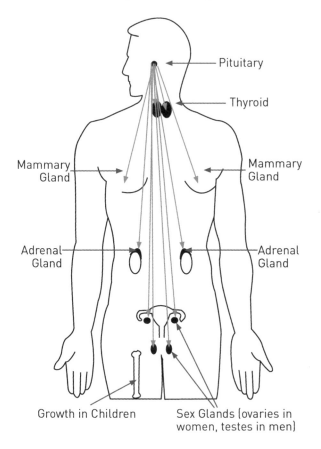

The pituitary gland: This gland controls many aspects of the endocrine system by sending messages to other glands to make more or less hormones.

I share the following information with you so you can truly marvel at, and deeply appreciate, what a miracle the human body really is. The pituitary gland actually functions as two separate compartments: the anterior (front) portion and the posterior (back) portion. The anterior pituitary is made up of a separate collection of individual cells that act as individual factories (termed "functional units") that are dedicated to produce a specific regulatory hormone messenger or factor. These factors are secreted in response to the outside environment and the internal bodily responses to this environment. These pituitary factors travel into the bloodstream and eventually reach their specific target gland. There, they stimulate the target gland to produce the appropriate type and amount of hormone so that the body can respond to the environment correctly. Isn't that absolutely amazing?

There are factories for a number of specific hormones, including cortisol, growth hormone, prolactin (related mostly to lactation, but can also be elevated in certain reproductive conditions, as discussed in the Beautiful Sex Hormones chapter), gonadotropin (stimulates the gonads), and one for thyroid-related stimulation. These five factories function as the anterior pituitary gland neuroendocrine unit. Again, no need to worry about any of these long-winded scientific names, I simply want you to see that the pituitary is the master controller of the endocrine glands we have explored in previous sections.

The posterior part of the pituitary stores and secretes hormones made by the hypothalamus. Both sections of the pituitary are directly connected to, and controlled by, the hypothalamus, a section of the brain controlling the basic survival processes of hunger, thirst, sexual reproduction, and self-defence. As I mentioned before, it is the part of the brain that, 24/7, asks the question: "Am I safe?" A stem containing both neurons (the nervous system) and small blood vessels (to transport the hormones of the endocrine system) connects the pituitary gland with the hypothalamus. Therefore, the hypothalamus communicates with the pituitary in two ways: by nerve impulses and by chemical messengers (hormones). The anterior pituitary receives instructions from the hypothalamus in the form of "releasing hormones". These chemical messengers produced by the hypothalamus then travel through the blood. A special network of vessels directs this blood through the anterior pituitary. In contrast, the posterior pituitary receives its messages through neural tissue and is controlled by nerve impulses.

If any one of the factories in the anterior part of the pituitary becomes excited and starts to overproduce its respective hormonal factor, the result is excess production of the final hormone product. For example, if the cortisol cells, called corticotrophs, lose their ability to respond to the normal stimuli from the environment, and from the hypothalamus, and develop their own independent, uncontrolled autonomous secretion, they will produce more cortisol than the body requires. In return, the adrenal glands will be overstimulated and secrete unregulated and unneeded stress chemicals, called catecholamines. The net result is excess production of these important chemicals that can signal fat storage, affect blood pressure (usually elevate it), and drive the heart rate higher, among other things. This can cause the body and internal organs to be stressed when there is no need. Unfortunately, the consequences of overdriving the internal organs of the body can take a toll on your health and, eventually, be life-threatening. In extreme cases, the cells that overproduce their respective hormones can clump together within a given area of the pituitary gland, creating a true factory of overproduction that would be diagnosed as a pituitary tumour. Not all pituitary tumours are cancerous; however, all tumours need medical attention due to the hormonal dysregulation they promote.

THE PITUITARY HORMONES

The pituitary gland makes six hormones from the anterior part and two from the posterior part. The **anterior lobe** makes:

- *thyroid stimulating hormone (TSH)* — signals the thyroid gland to make thyroid hormones
- *lutenizing hormone (LH)* — signals the ovaries
- *follicle stimulating hormone (FSH)* — signals the ovaries

- *prolactin* — stimulates breast development and breast milk production
- *growth hormone* — for the growth of all tissues in the body
- *adrenocorticotrophic hormone (ACTH)* — signals to the adrenals to make cortisol.

The **posterior lobe** makes:

- *antidiuretic hormone (ADH)* — controls how much urine is passed
- *oxytocin* — asks the uterus to contract at appropriate times in life (such as during childbirth and orgasm).

There are other endocrine glands in the body that do not need the pituitary gland to give them messages to produce their hormones. These glands include the parathyroids for calcium regulation and the pancreas for insulin production. They are controlled through other mechanisms.

To give you an example of how one of the pituitary hormones works, let's look at ACTH, whose job it is to direct the adrenal glands, whose function is essential to life. The hypothalamus produces an ACTH-releasing factor that stimulates ACTH secretion from the pituitary into the bloodstream. Specifically programmed receptors on the adrenal glands pick up the ACTH, and these receptors start sending signals to the centre of the cells (known as the cell nucleus) to start producing and secreting adrenal hormones. These hormones are then released into the circulatory system and their presence is communicated to the brain. The broad (family) names for some of the adrenal hormones include the glucocorticoids (such as cortisol), which influence the metabolism of the body, the mineralocorticoids (such as aldosterone), which are involved in regulating the amount of water in the body and hence blood pressure, and progesterone, which, as you know, is a hormone crucial to reproduction, as it prepares the uterus for the reception and preparation of a fertilized egg (ovum).

Like so many other hormones, ACTH is secreted in a circadian pattern over a 24-hour period. Each individual has their own internal circadian rhythm that determines how much sleep that person needs, when they are most alert, and when they prefer to eat. Disruptions of this rhythm can affect biological functions and moods, along with intellectual ability. For example, jet lag after a flight across a multitude of time zones is probably the result of a disruption of the circadian rhythm.

For most people, ACTH is at its highest blood level in the early morning and, with its action on the adrenals and the subsequent hormones that are produced, it influences whether you bounce or crawl out of bed. As the adrenals are the place from which we make our stress hormones, if stress goes on for too long some of the adrenals become less able to adapt to conditions. In other words, they get the message that they need to make stress hormones constantly when you may, in fact, be safe. This chronic stress pattern can deplete the adrenals over time, with chronic, deep fatigue as a typical symptom. (Although it is important to note that deep fatigue can be a symptom of many disorders.) Quite often with this health picture, the whole endocrine system needs support based on restorative practices, as outlined in the Beautiful Solutions chapter.

To really bring home to you just how extraordinary the body is, I want to share with you some biochemistry that totally spins my tyres. ACTH is actually a segment of a much larger glycoprotein prohormone molecule called proopiomelanocortin (POMC). A prohormone is a precursor to a hormone. Please don't worry about all of the whiz-bang scientific terms, just focus on the concept that follows.

POMC is synthesized by the corticotrophs of the anterior pituitary. POMC gets split into several biologically active polypeptides. Among these polypeptides is ACTH, whose major action is to stimulate the growth and secretion of the cells of the adrenal cortex. Other polypeptides derived from POMC include: melanocyte-stimulating hormone, specifically called alpha- and beta-melanotropin, which increase skin pigmentation; beta-lipotropin, which stimulates the release of fatty acid from adipose (fat) tissue; a small fragment of ACTH, which is believed to improve memory; and beta-endorphin, which suppresses pain. All that from one little prohormone!

When there is significant dysfunction with the pituitary gland, the following symptoms are common:

- headaches
- visual disturbances
- fatigue and lethargy
- inability to cope
- unexpected, abnormal, rapid growth (height)
- sleep disturbance
- nipple discharge
- impotence (men)
- absence or disturbance of the menstrual cycle
- skin and hair changes.

Not everyone will experience all of these symptoms or all at once. These signs and symptoms may occur because the target organ is not working effectively, and the pituitary gland itself may not be responsible. There are tests an endocrinologist can run to determine what precisely is going on. When there is a diagnosed pituitary condition, it will usually be necessary for an endocrinologist to prescribe replacement hormones.

SUBOPTIMAL PITUITARY FUNCTION (NO DISEASE)

I have seen countless women display symptoms that involve all or most of the organs that the pituitary governs without them having a full-blown pituitary condition. I call this suboptimal pituitary function. These women will display symptoms involving the adrenal glands (related to stress hormones), often the reproductive system (for example, PMS, PCOS, endometriosis, debilitating menopause), and sometimes the thyroid. If these women read information on the internet, they will say they can't work out if their problem is their adrenals, their sex hormones, or their thyroid, as they relate to the symptoms of dysfunction for each gland. They are usually tired but wired, and they rarely sleep well. Their moods change easily and unpredictably, and they are often impatient with or withdrawn from the people they love the most in this world. And then they berate themselves for being this way — hardly a winning formula for a happy life. If it is not clear to me, based on the symptoms, then I will test the stress hormones, the sex hormones, and thyroid function to get a clearer picture. What is apparent to me is that for so many women today, all three of these systems are affected, and not only do each of the affected glands need support, the pituitary does, too. I believe that for many this is the result of a subconscious fear: either a "fearful" state that their lifestyle choices, such as excess caffeine consumption, drive their body to perceive, or an emotional one, stemming from the belief (fear) that they are not (good) enough. I will explore this further in the Beautiful Insights chapter.

I meet countless women who tell me that they are

in love. And they are! And yet they are also in fear — fear that they will not do a good enough job, fear that they are not there enough for their children or friends, fear that their intimate relationship will end unless they are, or look, a certain way, fear that they will go broke, fear that they will get yelled at, fear that they don't look as good as they once did. Consequently, they do everything in their power to avoid ever having to feel that they are not enough, because it instinctively and subconsciously triggers their belief (fear) that if they aren't (good) enough, then they won't be loved. To prevent their fears from becoming realities, many women go into overdrive and get overwhelmed as they try to be all things to all people, which, for some, appears to lead to an overwhelmed state that takes its toll on the pituitary gland and the glands it controls.

CONTROL

Here's the "weirdo medicine" (an affectionate phrase used by colleagues) aspect of how I consider health conditions. If the pituitary gland is the control centre for the human body, then it seems logical to conclude that this gland will be particularly affected in women who describe themselves as "control freaks", women who have forgotten how to trust the unfolding of life, that each moment is all part of a bigger picture that we often can't see or understand. They have forgotten how to be fully present in each moment.

I was reminded recently of the joy we can, as adults, so easily miss. I was sitting on a park bench, watching people from all walks of life enjoy the sunshine and the outdoors. A mother threw a ball to her two sons (aged about eight and 10 years), one of whom had a developmental delay. This son didn't catch the ball every time she threw it to him, while her other son did. When the developmentally typical boy caught the ball, he had no change of expression on his face, or in his manner, and he simply threw the ball back to his mother. The boy with the developmental delay, however, celebrated every time he caught it! The delight and the excitement every time he caught the ball was as amped up as the first time he caught it, and he literally jumped with joy every time before he threw it back to his mother. Catching the ball had become routine to the younger, developmentally typical child, and he had lost his connection of glee to his ability, while the boy with the developmental delay was truly living in the moment and outwardly demonstrating how thrilled he was every time it happened.

How many of your own skills do you take for granted and no longer notice? Do you still pause at the feeling of human contact, someone else's skin on yours? Or the feeling of your pet's fur under your fingertips? Do you pause and breathe and tune in to how this feels? The first time you felt these things, it would have felt like magic to you. Pause long enough in each moment to experience the magic again. It is on offer 24/7. Only when we take our life for granted and tune out, when we rush, when we stand in front of the mirror bemoaning our [insert least favourite body part that you focus on] that we go momentarily blind. It is time to live your life in the light again and allow your pituitary gland to flourish.

AM I SAFE?

More and more, I am witnessing females of all ages face the following health picture. Your hypothalamus asks, 24/7: "Am I safe?" You don't realize it does this, but it has always done this. In doing so, it is assessing your physical environment. Is it too hot? Too cold? It is also asking this from an emotional perspective. Trouble is, you have beliefs that you don't even know you have. You create meanings from the looks on people's faces and the things they say, based on what you experienced as a child, whether you realize this or not. You think the world is how the world is, not how it really is, but *your* perceptions create *your* reality. You tell yourself stories constantly about who you are, and who and what you have to be in the world. And if based on the meanings you have set up in your nervous system your hypothalamus perceives that you are not safe (from being "yelled at" or "criticized", for example), then, without you knowing, it sends a message to the pituitary gland, which fires off the sympathetic nervous system and all of the necessary hormones so that you are ready to fight or flee. It throws you into the "red zone" I described earlier, and you then live from there.

That means the adrenals make adrenalin and/or cortisol, and most often both. Your adrenal production of progesterone is therefore decreased, meaning you lose this vital anti-anxiety agent, and oestrogen becomes dominant, which makes you fleshy, puffy, and kind of crazy. This means your thyroid gets a signal to either amp up or decrease its hormone production, and your blood glucose is not astutely regulated, which can lead you to feel like you want to eat your arm off, particularly sweet food. All of the above make it harder and harder to sleep well, further setting you up, biochemically, for your outer shine to fade from a lack of restoration — not to mention the stress it puts your insides. Not feeling safe feeds the cycle, and the chemistry that the cycle elicits keeps it going.

But when I spell it out like that, you can see where you may need to start to get your shine back to full glory … with your own mind. Of course I offer solutions for the various hormonal pictures I have described — that is a huge part of what I do and why people's health improves — and of course I will encourage you to step up and do all you can to give your body the opportunity to balance your sex hormones and stop churning out stress hormones, and reinvigorate your thyroid. There are many steps you can take to actively assist your body. Yet, at the same time, I strongly urge you to get to the heart of your matter, and see *why* you do what you do when you know what you know (let's face it, it's not a lack of education or knowledge that leads you to eat too much sugar — it's biochemical or emotional, or both!), or why you rush or feel overwhelmed, or why you don't feel safe. Otherwise it is like trying to stop a bath from overflowing by easing the plug out of the hole, while leaving the tap running. Exploring the emotional side of your health lets you to turn off the tap.

Real food fosters that exploration, that enquiry. It is very difficult to be kind, compassionate, and patient with others, or for you to even want to interact with people if you have a tendency to withdraw more, when you are filling yourself with stimulants and food that contain very little nutritional value. Choose real food that nourishes you, and watch your physical as well as your emotional health deeply radiate from within.

All I want for you right now at this stage in the book is to recognize the body systems that may need support, and for you to have an understanding of the power that real food, certain nutrients, and hydration play in your inner and outer health. Don't worry about your next step right now. Just recognize, with immense compassion for yourself, that it is what it is. The power to change your health is in your hands.

Tragically, there have been many disasters in the world of late, both natural (such as earthquakes) and domestic (such as violence), and when I talk about stress, I certainly do not want to make small of anything any of us may have been through. A natural disaster promotes the fight-or-flight response for a very good reason: to help you get out of danger and save your life. I know that for many thousands of women I have met who have been through such events that the stress continues long after the events themselves may have passed. If this applies to you, I admire your courage and resilience.

I offer you an article I wrote for a women's magazine after the earthquakes in Christchurch, New Zealand. Although some of the information you will have read in the Not-So-Beautiful Stress Hormones section, I left the article intact to reiterate the power of both human biochemistry and human hearts. And I also offer you the following thoughts. The impact and meaning of a catastrophe are not in the event itself. The ability to tolerate the event is a function not of what has occurred but of our relationship to our own minds and ourselves. In the simplicity of that realization is freedom.

The Stress Response

Given all that has happened in beautiful New Zealand recently, exploring ways health can be supported physically, mentally, and emotionally in times of stress is more important than ever. Firstly, let's examine what is going on inside the body in the aftermath of trauma and also the ongoing stress of what may be a deep worry about the future, experienced by many New Zealanders at this time.

Humans have extraordinary resilience, both mentally and physically, and the body has an innate capacity to heal. Remember that! We really are amazing. However, to assist that process, there is much we can do to support our body's stress response. Here, I describe the physicality of the stress response, not so that you worry more, but so that if your body, health, or mind-set starts to change you can rest assured that it is a natural process and that your body has an extraordinary capacity to heal.

Stage 1

Adrenalin is our acute stress hormone, the one that makes our heart race. It can make us shake, drive our thoughts to race, or make us jump when we are startled. It also stops our digestive system from working optimally, as adrenalin wants you to stay focused on whatever is threatening your life. Adrenalin puts us on "red alert", meaning we are geared to fight or flee. Initially, when we get a shock, this is the body's survival response, designed to get us out of danger.

Adrenalin is the initial, primary stress hormone made by anyone involved in, or directly affected by, *the recent earthquakes. Some people get biochemically stuck in this state because the fear of another earthquake, or concerns for family, continue psychologically. Sleep can then be affected, since your body perceives that your life is in danger. If you sleep deeply, your body worries that you won't be ready to fight or flee. The best tactic on the planet to calm yourself from this state is to change your focus to something for which you are grateful, and I don't say that flippantly. And shift your breathing back into a pattern that makes your belly move in and out with each breath, rather than your chest. Nothing communicates to your nervous system that you are safe better than diaphragmatic breathing.*

There are also herbs that can assist you in recovering from a stressful event, and these include withania, passionflower, and zizyphus. Keeping hydrated is also essential, as is additional vitamin B, found in whole grains (if your digestion tolerates them), vitamin C, found in many fruits, and capsicum and magnesium, found in green leafy vegetables and nuts.

Stage 2

After the initial shock, the second stage of stress is typically initiated. This involves the production of a different stress hormone called cortisol, which historically humans only produced in excess during floods, famines, or wars; all times when food was scarce. As a result of this, cortisol often makes you eat too much food, because when food abounds, your cortisol-fuelled body thinks you are so lucky to have found a whole packet of crackers! Sleep is affected in this state, too; however, this poor sleep generally means you fall asleep OK but you wake between 2am and 3am, when cortisol naturally rises. Cortisol initially does wonderful things for the body in this state of stress, as it is a powerful anti-inflammatory. We need the anti-inflammatory action to protect us from the metabolic inflammation adrenalin can cause. The problem for our health is that when the stress goes on too long for the body to handle — this threshold is different for everyone — cortisol starts to break down your muscles, suppress your immune system, and make your desire for sweet food almost uncontrollable. Excellent ways to support yourself through a period of elevated cortisol include doing diaphragmatic breathing exercises daily, doing "yin" exercise, such as restorative yoga or t'ai chi, using herbs, such as Siberian ginseng, rhodiola, licorice, or withania, and filling your diet with as many fresh foods as you can.

Stage 3

The next biochemical stage of stress that can occur, especially if the stress has been prolonged, may involve cortisol falling low. If you have had a high level of cortisol output for many, many years, your adrenal glands may not be able to stand the tension and so they "crash". In general terms, you burn out. In more recent times, this has become known as adrenal fatigue, because the major symptom at this stage is an unrelenting, deep fatigue.

Cortisol is supposed to be high in the morning, and ideal amounts help you bounce out of bed. It plays a role in how vital you feel and helps the body combat any inflammatory processes that want to kick in. Stiffness is a key symptom of adrenal fatigue. For those with chronic stress, morning cortisol levels tend to be low; it can be very difficult to get out of bed with such low levels, which in itself can lead you to feel flat in your mood as well. By mid-afternoon, it will be at an all-time low, and you feel you need something sweet, something containing caffeine, or a nap to get you through your afternoon. For an adrenally fatigued person, cortisol is nice and low in the evenings, but if you don't go to bed before 10pm, you will typically get a second wind, and it will be much harder for you to fall asleep if you are still up at midnight. The fatigue you feel with this biochemical picture may make exercise the least appealing thing on the planet to you. You actually feel worse after exercise when you are adrenally fatigued, whereas exercise typically energizes. For people with deep, deep fatigue, I almost always use the following herbal tonic that contains:

- *panex ginseng*
- *licorice*
- *dandelion leaves*
- *astragalus*
- *one other herb depending on what else is going for the individual (a liver herb or a reproductive herb are typical).*

I also sometimes use a range of supplements from the United States, created by Dr James Wilson, specifically for adrenal fatigue. I have had countless clients *take this range of supplements for three months and have their energy and vitality return to great levels.*

Humans were never designed to sustain long-term stress, and our individual bodies cope with it in different ways. For some, adrenalin remains the dominant stress hormone all of their life, while others may flip over into a more cortisol-dominant stress response. If the stress response doesn't truly switch off, there is the potential that the adrenals will eventually crash, and cortisol output is no longer optimum or elevated; instead, it is negligible. At its extreme, this condition is called Addison's disease. Yet if a person has an extremely low cortisol level but that level still falls just inside the "normal" range, that person will be told that they are fine. They feel lousy, yet all of the tests they have always come back "normal". They feel anything but normal, and people who know and love them will often comment that they are a shell of their former selves.

Long-term, cortisol can also be rather sinister in that it can interfere with your sex hormone metabolism, your sleep patterns via its interference with melatonin, and also your mood via serotonin.

Real Food

Although I often recommend supplements of herbs and/or nutrients during times of stress, never underestimate the healing and restorative power of food the way it comes in Nature. Taking supplements is not a reason to eat a poor-quality, low-nutrient diet. I simply recommend supplements where appropriate and especially to assist in the restoration of health.

Finally, human kindness goes a long way towards healing, and we have been privileged to witness extraordinary acts of compassion in the aftermath of the earthquakes. The courage of this nation is spectacular.

~~~~~~~~~~~~~~~~~~

*We are all a little weird and life's a little weird,
and when we find someone whose weirdness is
compatible with ours, we join up with them and fall
in mutual weirdness and call it love.*

Dr Seuss

Chapter 5
Beautiful Detox:
how the liver and elimination
pathways support your shine

When it comes to health and beauty, the liver packs a mighty punch. It is one of the big guns when it comes to your skin, your eyes, your hormonal balance, and your vitality. In conjunction with the gallbladder, the liver works endlessly to help us excrete fatty substances that the body no longer needs, including old hormones, pesticides, as well as stored body fat.

The liver is the body's second largest organ after our skin. It sits behind your right ribcage. Its primary role is detoxification, a concept that has had much confusion surrounding it — confusion I want to resolve for you!

A simple way to imagine the detoxification power of the liver is to picture a triangle shape: inside that triangle are billions and billions of little circles, each one of them a liver cell. Imagine that inside each liver cell is a mouse on a wheel, running and running and running, with each turn of the billions of little wheels driving your liver function. When we treat our liver unkindly, a circle can die, and, for a while, the liver can regenerate a new cell to replace the dead cell, but, after a while this is no longer possible, and a globule of fat can take up residence where once that fat-burning little "mouse" was working.

When many fat globules take over (known as "fatty liver"), our health and our appearance can suffer. A less efficient detox processes can lead to poor skin quality, poor thyroid function, sex hormone imbalances, lousy cholesterol, and impaired blood glucose management that often shows up as sugar cravings. Moreover, where our body wants to lay down body fat can also shift. For the first time people may notice that they have a fat roll quite high up on their abdomen. For women, this is just below their bra and, for men, just beneath their pectoral muscles. It can come and go, and sometimes there is a point right in the centre of the torso that is tender. I will always suggest ways to support your liver based on the presence of a fat roll in that position, and gallbladder support based on that tender point. Sometimes both organs need support. In the not-too-distant past, only people who regularly over-consumed alcohol developed fatty liver disease, but now we are seeing teenagers develop it simply from eating diets high in processed foods.

DETOXIFICATION

There are numerous organs and body systems involved in detoxification. They include:

- the *liver* — your first line of defence against toxins, it acts like a filter, preventing the toxic substances contained in foods and the environment from passing into your blood

- the *colon* (digestive system) — it contains bacteria that produce both healthy and unhealthy chemicals, so you want to keep your bowel moving regularly, as its main role is to flush out toxic chemicals so they don't accumulate

- the *kidneys* — they are constantly filtering your blood and getting rid of anything you don't need, including toxins, in the form of urine

- the *skin* — not only does it protect and house your organs, but toxins are able to leave the body via perspiration

- the *respiratory system* — even the hairs inside your nose help filter the air you breathe in — while many people don't consider the lungs as a part of your detoxification squad, they are responsible for filtering out fumes, allergens, mould, and airborne toxins; when we are stressed, we tend to shift from slow belly breathing to short, shallow upper chest breaths, which in turn can reduce the lungs' ability to transport oxygen to all tissues; for those of you who know my work, you now know another reason (other than the nervous system and stress-hormone-lowering benefits) why diaphragmatic breathing is my number one health tip.

Detoxification is a process that goes on inside us all day, every day. The choices we make influence how efficiently the liver is able to do its job. Detoxification is essentially a transformation process. Any substance that would be harmful to you if it accumulated in your body must be changed into a less harmful form so that it can then be excreted safely from your body. To look and feel your best, you want this to be a highly efficient process.

There are two stages to the detoxification process, appropriately named phase 1 and phase 2 liver detoxification. Both stages require certain nutrients to function, and dietary choices can influence how efficiently each phase is able to work. The figure below

illustrates the phases of detoxification, and you can
see some of the nutrients that are required.

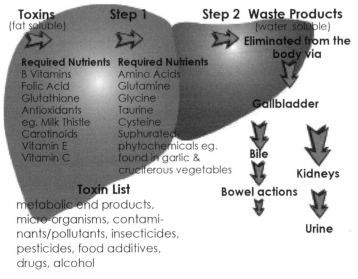

Liver detoxification pathways: Phase 1 and phase 2 liver
detoxification pathways, and the nutrients essential to these
vital processes.

Phase 1

For the first stage of detoxification, numerous nutrients, including B vitamins, are essential. Whole grains
are one of the richest sources of B vitamins we have
in the food supply; however, many people feel much
better with fewer or none of these foods in their diets.
People decrease or cut grains out of their diets for
varied reasons. Some first experienced rapid weight
loss with the advent of the high-protein, very low-
carbohydrate diets, purported as the ultimate answer
to weight-loss desires in the late 1990s, a repeat of the

popular dietary concept from the 1970s, and a natural progression from the high-carbohydrate, super-low-fat guidelines that had preceded them. Others simply started to notice that foods made from grains induced reflux or made their tummy bloated, and they took action to change how they felt. If grains feel good for you and energize you, then enjoy them in whole food form; some are best soaked prior to consumption. If they don't suit you, don't eat them. Your body knows best what works for you. Simply be aware that if you have a low intake of B vitamins, your phase 1 liver detoxification processes may not function optimally. It can be useful to take a supplement if you eat a low-carbohydrate diet or avoid/limit grains.

Phase 2

There is one road into the liver and five pathways out of the liver. Just as for phase 1 reactions, phase 2 liver pathways also require certain nutrients to function, in particular, specific amino acids and sulphur.

We get our amino acids from protein foods. Really think about this next statement. What we eat becomes part of us. Protein foods are broken down into amino acids, and they go on to create all of the cells of your immune system, which are what defends you from infection. Amino acids also go on to create the neurotransmitters in your brain that influence your mood and clarity of thought. They also build your pretty muscles that allow you to carry your groceries. What you eat really does matter — your food becomes part of you.

Phase 2 pathways use, among other substances, amino acids and sulphur. We obtain sulphur from eggs, onion, garlic, and shallots, as well as from the *Brassica* family of vegetables, which includes broccoli, cabbage, kale, Brussels sprouts, and cauliflower. The liver makes enzymes that are responsible for the transformation of each substance, and the rate of production of these essential enzymes determines how quickly each substance is processed. The load placed on the liver also determines how quickly things move through the liver, and you will see shortly how all of this impacts on how you look and feel, particularly on your skin.

Liver Loaders

There is a group of substances I lovingly label "liver loaders". Can you guess what they are? They include:

- alcohol
- caffeine
- trans fats
- refined sugars
- synthetic substances (for example, pesticides, medications, skin "care")
- infection (for example, viruses such as glandular fever — Epstein-Barr virus, mononucleosis).

As outlined in the Beautiful Foods chapter, when we consider our exposure to synthetic substances we must consider skin care. We are crazy if we think that we don't absorb things through our skin. You only have to look at the way nicotine patches work to realize that the skin is a quick and easy route from our skin to our blood stream, carrying the blood that the liver will need to clean. There are plenty of wonderful skin-care companies out there who do not use synthetic ingredients. Seek them out or even make your own. I love to suggest to people that it would be good if they could eat their skin care! You want to be able to recognise the words on the label of your skin care, just as you do with food.

It is not, however, just infections, or the things we consume or put on our skin that can place demands on the detoxification processes of the liver. Substances your body makes itself also need transformation by the liver so that they can be excreted. These substances include:

- cholesterol
- steroid hormones, such as oestrogen
- substances created by or causing any shortfall in digestion, due to compromised digestive processes, as explored in the Beautiful Digestion chapter
- untreated food sensitivities
- undiagnosed coeliac disease.

I have met countless people who have not consumed much in the way of liver loaders, but have diabolical menstrual cycles or an ongoing challenge with irritable bowel syndrome or constipation, and often exhibit what I consider to be distinct signs that their liver needs support. Passing clots while menstruating is a classic liver congestion sign, as are most skin conditions. More signs are listed below.

INDICATIONS YOUR LIVER NEEDS SUPPORT

The following are signs that may indicate that your liver needs support:

- liver roll
- a tender point in the centre of your torso (which can indicate gallbladder issues, past emotional heartbreak, or massive disappointment); if your gallbladder has been removed, your liver has to make the bile the gallbladder once did, so additional liver support is often required
- short fuse or bad temper
- episodes or feelings of intense anger
- "liverish", gritty, impatient behaviour
- premenstrual syndrome
- cellulite (lymphatic or cortisol related also)
- congested skin or skin outbreaks related to the menstrual cycle
- skin rashes

- eczema, rosacea
- overheating easily
- "floaters" in your vision (can also be a sign of iron deficiency)
- waking around 2am
- poor sleep on an evening you consume alcohol
- waking up hot during the night
- not hungry for breakfast when you first get up in the morning
- preference for coffee to start your day
- elevated cholesterol
- oestrogen-dominance symptoms
- bloating easily
- daily alcohol consumption
- daily long-term caffeine consumption.

Cholesterol

Cholesterol is an extremely important substance. We only ever hear bad press about cholesterol; however, we would melt without it. It is the building block of all of our steroid hormones, including progesterone and testosterone. The process that cholesterol undergoes to form steroid hormones is illustrated in the diagram below.

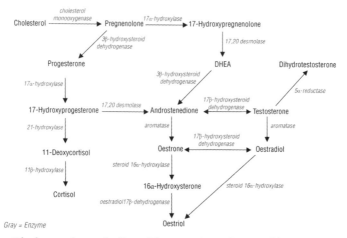

Cholesterol metabolism: The creation of steroid hormones from cholesterol.

The reason I include the above biochemical diagram is to literally illustrate the way substances in the body flow onward to create other substances. Only some of the cholesterol that the body makes, or that you obtain from your diet, remains as cholesterol. You do not want too much cholesterol accumulating as cholesterol; you want it to turn into progesterone, testosterone, DHEA, and oestrogen. All of the words in the diagram that begin with "Oest" are different forms of oestrogen.

Your diet contributes to approximately 20 per cent of the amount of cholesterol in your blood, while your liver creates the other 80 per cent. Your liver makes cholesterol when it needs to protect itself, as, in such situations, cholesterol behaves like an anti-inflammatory. What are some of the things that may inflame the liver and drive additional cholesterol production? The liver loaders listed above! One of the most successful ways to manage your blood level of cholesterol is to take extra good care of your liver and deal with any inflammation in the body with a good-quality essential fat supplement. To illustrate the immense power of your liver: there is not one person in 15 years whose cholesterol I haven't lowered back into the normal range simply by guiding them to take care of their liver. Over time, I have also been able to witness the other incredible health and beauty benefits that unfold when we focus on taking care of our liver. For me, elevated cholesterol is simply one way the body communicates that the liver needs some additional support.

Healthy cholesterol metabolism is best imagined as a gently flowing stream. You want a small amount of cholesterol to remain in your blood as cholesterol, but you want the majority of the cholesterol to be converted into your sex (also sometimes referred to as steroid) hormones. Men and women make all three of the major sex hormones, specifically testosterone, oestrogen, and progesterone. Each sex makes them in differing ratios, with men producing more testosterone and far less oestrogen along with some progesterone, while women make more oestrogen and progesterone and less testosterone. You can see from the diagram that certain enzymes push the hormones one way or the other. Sometimes over time, however, too much cholesterol can accumulate as cholesterol. To come back to the analogy of cholesterol metabolism being like a flowing stream, it is as though a dam wall gets built across the flow and, instead of cholesterol being converted into sex hormones, it accumulates in the blood as cholesterol. There are two problems here.

One is that too much blood cholesterol may pose a health problem. Although, the jury is still out on whether this is actually true from a heart disease perspective; my opinion is that cholesterol is not related to heart disease, and science is starting to show that the original conclusions drawn from the research linking cholesterol and heart disease were most likely incorrect. Cholesterol is only a problem in your blood if the wall of a blood vessel is damaged by a free radical, which occurs if there aren't enough antioxidants present to pair up with the free radical, or if there is elevated blood glucose, as this leads cholesterol to become sticky and act like a plaster covering and protecting the site of the damage. The other is that you now have lower levels of sex hormones being produced. Your steroid hormones make you feel vital and alive. They are an enormous contributing factor to whether you bounce or stagger out of bed each morning, and whether your skin is free from blemishes, and glows. When your sex hormones are balanced and at optimal levels, you feel amazing.

For cholesterol to be converted into sex hormones, you must have great zinc levels; essential fatty acids are also important. Our best sources of the omega-3 fats are the oils in fish, flaxseeds (linseeds), walnuts, and pecans, while evening primrose oil and borage oil are good sources of the essential fats of the omega-6 type. The richest food source of zinc is oysters. Beef and lamb also contain some, and our vegetable sources include seeds, such as sunflower seeds and pumpkin seeds. So far as amounts go, however, oysters contain 70 milligrams of zinc per 100 grams, while beef, being the next best source of zinc, contains only 4 milligrams. Lamb has on average 2.9 milligrams of zinc, while seeds have around 0.9 milligrams of zinc per 100 grams. In the not-so-distant past, we obtained consistent amounts of zinc from our plant foods. But food is only as good as the quality of the soil, and if a nutrient is not in the soil, then it cannot be in our food! Most soil in the Western world is deficient in zinc unless it has been organically or — better still from a zinc perspective — biodynamically farmed. Each adult needs a minimum of 15 milligrams of zinc per day just so the body can perform its basic functions. That is potentially not even enough for optimal health. So from where on Earth are we getting our zinc? The answer is that many of us are not. Studies have suggested that approximately 70 per cent of people living in Western countries are deficient in zinc, and it is a mineral that is not only essential for keeping cholesterol levels in check and producing optimal amounts of sex hormones, but is also vital to our skin health and wound healing, as well as digestion and immune function. Zinc is a mighty little mineral!

The second part of this biochemical picture about cholesterol metabolism and liver health involves the excretion of cholesterol. The same mechanism also applies to oestrogen, so for any female who read the previous section about sex hormones and identified oestrogen dominance in her life, this is incredibly important.

When a liver loader, either consumed (exogenous) or made as a result of internal chemistry (endogenous), arrives at the front door of the liver, it has arrived to be transformed. So when any of the liver loaders (in this case, let's remain focused on cholesterol) arrive at the front door of the liver, they undergo their first stage of change (phase 1 liver detoxification). Between the front door and the middle of the liver, cholesterol is still cholesterol, but it has been altered somewhat. This slightly changed cholesterol then wants to go down one of the five phase 2 detox roads, and, once it has done that, it has been slightly altered again, and it is this substance that can then be excreted — gone from your body forever.

Health problems can arise, however, when the traffic on the phase 2 pathways gets all banked up like traffic on a motorway. After years of regularly consumed liver loaders, and/or hormonal or bowel problems, the roads out of the liver can become congested. Conventional blood tests for liver function do not reveal this. The liver usually takes years of battering before conventional blood tests reflect the congestion that led to them becoming elevated in the first place. When the traffic is banked up, the cholesterol, or oestrogen, undergoes its first stage of change and arrives in the middle of the liver, ready to go down its appropriate path for the second stage of transformation it must undergo before it can be excreted. If the phase 2 pathways are congested, the cholesterol (or oestrogen) sitting in the middle of the liver has nowhere to go, and it cannot remain waiting in the middle of the liver as there is more rubbish constantly coming through the front door of the liver. When this happens, the liver then releases the cholesterol, or oestrogen, back out into the blood, where it gets recycled. It is the recycling of these substances, not the substances themselves, which is potentially harmful to human health. What organ can we take much better care of if we want to stop this recycling from happening? Our precious liver. Our livers need more love, and less of a load, for health and shine, inside and out.

On another note, remember that it is the recycled form of oestrogen that is of such concern for women regarding the risk of developing reproductive cancers, as discussed in the chapter on sex hormones. Oestrogen is a beautiful hormone in the right amount and with the right types of oestrogen being dominant. Too much total oestrogen or too much of the wrong type are the problems, because of the oestrogen itself and also because progesterone production can never match it. The liver is involved in countless mechanisms linked to beauty so be sure to read some of the additional free blog posts at: www.drlibby.com/bioresources

ANTIOXIDANT DEFENCE MECHANISMS

Another way the body detoxifies, other than through phase 1 and 2 detoxification pathways, is through our antioxidant defence mechanisms. This is a superb aspect of our chemistry, and, although we looked at it in Beautiful Foods, it is so important that it is worth revisiting here. Humans stay alive through a process called respiration, meaning that we breathe in oxygen, and we exhale carbon dioxide. If you could see oxygen in space, it is two Os (oxygen molecules) stuck together. The diagram on page 50 illustrates what is described here.

When we breathe, oxygen splits apart, forming two single oxygen molecules. Known as free radicals, they have the potential to damage your tissues. One of the major ways the body defends itself from damage by a free radical is through the consumption of antioxidants. Antioxidant-rich foods are our coloured plant foods. Blueberries, green tea, red wine, and chocolate (cacao) are rich in antioxidants, and are the most common antioxidant-rich foods called out at my live events when I ask the audience for ideas. As the skins and seeds of the red grapes are especially high in antioxidants, grape juice is just as powerful as red wine (from an antioxidant perspective), and doesn't ask the liver to do extra detox work. The antioxidant donates one of its oxygens back to the free radical, and they pair up. Oxygen is then content again, and damage to your tissues is avoided.

To understand one powerful way free radicals can damage our tissues, imagine a blood vessel leading to your heart. A free radical zips about through the blood and suddenly does a dive-bomb and makes an indentation in the wall of the vessel. It resembles the divot in the grass beneath a golf swing that has taken too much soil with it. The damaged vessel sends out a cry for help, signalling that it is damaged, and, in this case, cholesterol wants to be the hero. Cholesterol behaves like a band-aid in this situation, and it comes along and sticks itself on top of the injured site. It then sends out a message to all of its cholesterol friends to join the band-aid party, and they come along and stick themselves over the top of the first cholesterol globule that arrived. The cholesterol piles up, and it oxidises and hardens. This is called atherosclerosis or plaque, and it narrows the interior of the arteries. Where once the blood could flow through a wide, open vessel, it now has a very narrow, restricted path to weave. Your blood is the only way oxygen and nutrients get around your body. Your heart is a muscle, and it needs both oxygen and nutrients to survive. If it is starved of either of these for long enough, it can lead to a heart attack.

The good news, though, is that this condition is reversible. The hardened, built-up cholesterol is LDL cholesterol, which is why it is commonly known as "bad" cholesterol. "Good" cholesterol (HDL cholesterol) comes along and unsticks each globule of cholesterol and carries it off to — guess where? You guessed it: the liver. It arrives at the front door of the liver to undergo its detoxification process and, when the liver is functioning well, the cholesterol is processed, excreted, and gone forever. However, as outlined previously, if the liver is loaded up with substances that it *must* prioritize higher up the detox order than boring old, homemade cholesterol, then the cholesterol reaches the midpoint of the liver, gets released too soon, and gets reabsorbed. And that is one major way our blood cholesterol goes up and up and up. Cholesterol can also be elevated when thyroid function is poor.

I cannot conclude talking about liver detoxification

without talking about liver loader number one, alcohol. There's a reason it is at the top of the list — I consider it one of the most pervasive substances impacting too many livers today. I see people who might eat as green as can be, but at the same time consume alcohol daily. Alcohol is certainly a substance that can take away our shine and sometimes the shine of others, particularly when it is regularly over-consumed. As a society, we need to get real about the dangers of routine alcohol consumption. Here is an article I wrote for the post-holiday season.

Alcohol

As the festive season draws to a close, the effects of too much alcohol may still be silently, or loudly, reverberating. Whether it is increased body fat or cellulite, less energy, worse bouts of PMS, or mood fluctuations . . . or perhaps your get up and go has got up and left, the price of over-consumption is just not worth it. As fun as it can be at the time, alcohol can rob you of your clarity and purpose. And so January often sees us making big statements about our health, alcohol reduction, or avoidance. Some wait until February to take a break, as they've worked out it has the least number of days! I know others who do Dry July in July or Oct-sober in October.

We drink for wide and varied reasons. For some, it is the way they socialise, or the way they wind down from the day. Some use alcohol to distract themselves from thoughts and feelings they'd rather avoid. It can be a way that people cope. Regardless of the reason, many of us overdrink without even realising it.

A standard drink is 100 grams of alcohol, in whatever form that comes. In Australia and New Zealand, 100 grams of alcohol is a 330-millilitre bottle of 4 per cent beer, a 30-millilitre nip of spirits, 170 millilitres of champagne, or a measly 100 millilitres of wine — about four swallows! Next time you pour yourself a glass of wine, measure it, and see what your natural pour is. For most, it is considerably more than 100 millilitres, and, as a result, many of us are overdrinking without even realising.

The current recommendations provided by heart foundations say that for women no more than two standard drinks per day with two alcohol-free days (AFDs) per week is OK, while, for men, three standard drinks per day and two AFDs is OK.

We have long heard the heart health benefits of red wine publicly sung, and, for some, this somehow justifies that drinking is OK — you are clearly looking after your heart. But I also encourage you to consider many of the cancer organisations from around the world's position statement on alcohol, which says that if you have a family history of cancer, there is no safe level of alcohol consumption … a very powerful statement to contemplate.

I'm not suggesting that you don't drink. Having a drink can be immensely pleasurable for those who partake on occasions. I simply want to appeal to you to get honest with yourself about how alcohol affects you. You know in your heart if you drink too much and when it is negatively impacting your *health. Alcohol can affect the way we relate to those we love the most in the world, and of course it affects how you feel about yourself. So, if you drink, drink for the pleasure of it or to celebrate, rather than to escape your life or due to the misconstrued message that alcohol is good for your health.*

The link between the consistent, overconsumption of alcohol and breast cancer is undeniable. Research has shown this time and time again and for many years now. Yet, we rarely hear about it.

The human body cannot excrete alcohol; it has to be converted into acetaldehyde by the liver, and then the acetaldehyde can be excreted. This is the nasty substance that can accumulate and give us a head-ache/hangover excessive consumption. If the liver doesn't do its job properly and alcohol accumulates in our blood, we can go into a coma and die. Alcohol is a poison to the human body and I don't say that lightly. But, thankfully, usually our liver jumps to action and starts the conversion process and we can carry on. Over time, though, this takes its toll.

When we drink daily, or, for some, just regularly, the liver can be so busy dealing with alcohol as its priority that other substances the liver has to change so they can be excreted don't get any attention and are recycled. Oestrogen and cholesterol are two examples. It is often the reabsorption of these substances that leads to elevated levels in our body, and that can lead to health challenges.

If you want to cut back or cut out alcohol for a while, or even if you just want to break your habit of regular drinking, still pour yourself a drink at the time you would normally have a glass of wine, and do what you would normally do. Sit and chat to your partner, make dinner, talk on the phone to a friend. So often we have mentally linked the glass of wine to a pleasurable activity when it is actually the pleasurable activity that we don't want to miss out on! So have sparkling water in a wine glass, with some fresh lime or lemon if that appeals, and add a few more AFDs to your life.

~~~~~~~~~~~~~~~~~~~~

BEAUTY FOCUS

When it comes to your skin and your sparkle, one of the first places I focus is on great liver health. If the liver is unable to make its enzymes fast enough to detoxify the substances that your body perceives is a problem for it (whether these substances are from outside the body or being made within the body), the body may utilize another detoxification process, which is essentially excretion through the skin. The skin may be inflamed in some way or it may be congested. There may be break-outs or cystic pimples.

With these signs, digestive system support and/or dietary change will almost always be highly beneficial. When you pause to think about it, you absorb all of the goodness, all of the nutrients, out of your food in your digestive system, and the nutrients move from here across and into your blood. That is how you are nourished. So if your food is of poor quality, meaning that it is devoid of most nutrients, or if it contains substances that may actually take away from your health, such as artificial sweeteners, additives, or preservatives, all of your "beauty bits" may not be getting the fuel they need to shine. For example, if there isn't enough calcium being eaten and absorbed (caffeine blocks calcium absorption), then your nails have little chance of being lovely.

Furthermore, excellent elimination also plays a vital role in many aspects of our appearance. The whites of the eyes tend to be more on the bloodshot side when digestion and/or the liver need some support. Using your bowels daily, or twice daily, is very healthy and is the main passage of waste out of the body. One of the best ways to support optimal elimination is through eating a diet high in real food, particularly plants. Your body knows how to digest real food. I cannot guarantee that it knows what to do with man-made "food".

It may be time for some liver love! Here are some ideas to take your liver support to the next level.

Liver-loving Solutions and Ideas

Set yourself a time-based goal when it comes to making these changes. For example: "I will drink alcohol only on weekends for four weeks" or "I will drink coffee only when I go out for breakfast on Sundays." Here are some options to get you started:

- take a break from alcohol

- drink only on weekends

- replace coffee with green or white tea (or, less often, weak, black tea), or swap all hot drinks to herbals (no caffeine)

- take beneficial liver herbs such as:

    o St Mary's thistle, especially if alcohol is a regular part of your life

    o globe artichoke, especially of you have a tendency to constipation and/or a liver roll and/or central torso tenderness

    o bupleurum, especially if you have clots in the menstrual blood

    o schisandra, especially for its detox action (it also works on the adrenals)

- transform anger into passion by giving a different meaning to a past experience

    o the energy of anger and passion are the same, but they manifest in vastly different ways — one ignites, the other often extinguishes

- resolve any underlying anger that may, or may not, be quite silent and unexpressed —

in numerous traditional medicine systems, the liver is the seat of anger in the body, and can be expressed in long-term skin challenges

- o understand that anger may be a sign that your needs are not being met and work to alter this
- drink vegetable juice or a green smoothie each morning
- snack on seeds and nuts
- consume less fruit and none after morning tea
- cut out dairy products for a four-week trial, and/or
- cut out grains containing gluten for a four-week trial
- consider an essential fatty acid supplement, and consider a higher dose if cholesterol is elevated
- consume high-zinc foods such as oysters (from clean waters), or take a zinc supplement of zinc picolinate, 15–30 milligrams per day, best taken at night just before bed to maximize absorption.

Remember, it is what you do every day that impacts on your health, not what you do sometimes. Be honest with yourself about the liver loaders in your life. And take such good care of yourself that you can deeply experience how beautiful your inner world and your outer world truly are. We only have one liver. Love it accordingly.

Scatter sunshine.

Dr Libby

Chapter 6
Beautiful Digestion:
the basis of beauty

When making changes to optimize your health and beauty, improving your digestion is a key place to start. We all know that it is best to build your house on a strong foundation, and building a robust digestive system is much the same. Gut issues are widespread, with one in five women in many Western countries reportedly suffering from irritable bowel syndrome (IBS). You only have to look at the amount of advertising targeted at improving gut health to see the prevalence of this problem. Improving digestion can have the most profound effect on your overall health and appearance. With simple, easy steps, you can make radical changes.

It never ceases to amaze me how magnificent and how clever our bodies really are, and it astounds me how many processes go on inside the body without us having to give them any thought. Digestion is one of those processes, and it is central to our beauty; it is the way we get all of the goodness out of our food, and the nourishment we get as result of good digestion is an extraordinary gift without which we would not survive. Digestion is intricate and complex, and yet relatively robust. And it is intimately connected to how you feel and function every single day, from your energy level to the fat you burn, from the texture and appearance of your skin to whether you have a bloated tummy, right down to your mood. Digestion is responsible for so much that goes on inside us. If it is a body system that gives you grief, if you are bloated most evenings, if you have intermittent diarrhoea and constipation, or if you get reflux, you can reach a point where you feel like that is how life is always going to be. It must just be how you are. Perhaps you believe it is "in the family". Well, bowel challenges do *not* have to be your reality.

Digestion is the perfect, and actually the first, place to start for amazing health and when you want to solve any beauty challenge. It can be a challenge to balance hormones, for example, if your digestion is the bane of your life. Likewise, if the gut is not working optimally, it will often show up in the skin, as the skin is just another pathway of elimination for the body. Some of the information in this section may make you giggle ... it can be a challenge to find the right words to describe our stools! And some of the advice may at first seem obvious and too simple to make much of a difference. But reflect on your own eating habits and digestive system functions as you read on, and be ready to take your well-being and sparkle to whole new level!

HOW THE DIGESTIVE SYSTEM WORKS

Digestion sustains us. It is the process of breaking down food so that we can absorb and utilise it for energy and to sustain our lives. Food is simply broken down into smaller components. For example, proteins are broken down into amino acids, and it is through this breakdown of food, and our absorption of these smaller substances, that we are nourished.

The digestive system is made up of a digestive tract, a big, long tube (imagine it looking like a hose), and numerous ancillary organs, including the liver, gallbladder, and pancreas. The following illustration gives you an idea. The big, long tube begins at your mouth, moves down the oesophagus, through a valve, and into your stomach. The food then moves through a valve at the bottom side of the stomach and into the small intestine, through the small intestine and ileocaecal valve into the large intestine, and then any waste is excreted out the other end. When this process works well, you look and feel fantastic. When it is in any way impaired, the opposite can be true, and correcting it can change your life.

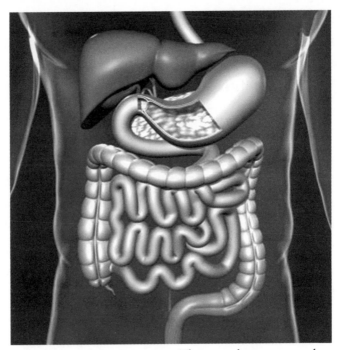

The human digestive system: The oesophagus enters the stomach (a cut-away section is shown above). The tube continues into the small intestine (the smooth tube above) and then into the large intestine (the indented tube section above). Finally, the waste is excreted. The liver is shown high on the left, the gallbladder in tucked in underneath the liver on the left, and the pancreas appears to sit behind the stomach pouch in the centre of the upper third of the image.

SUPPORTING DIGESTION

Chew Your Food

Food enters the mouth and moves down the oesophagus into the stomach. But what do we do to our food before it reaches the stomach? We chew it — or, in some cases, inhale it! There are no more teeth beyond the mouth: you can't chew food once it has left your mouth. Yet so many people eat as though their oesophagus is lined with teeth. Many of us are in such a hurry with our meals, or we are so excited by the flavour of our food, that we might chew each mouthful four times if we are lucky. It's a case of chew, chew, chew, chew, mmmmm yum, next forkful in, chew, chew, oh gosh my mouth is so full, better swallow some food ... so we swallow some partially chewed food and some not-at-all-chewed food, and we do this day in, day out, year after year. And somehow we expect our stomach just to cope. This alone can be the basis of digestive system problems, such as bloating, that appear further along the tract.

The stomach gets to a point where it doesn't like the rules by which you are playing anymore, so it takes its bat and goes home. So, slow down! Chew your food! If you are a food inhaler, try this: put food into your mouth, chew it really well, and then swallow it before you put the next mouthful in. I know that sounds simple, but try it. It can take an enormous amount of concentration for food inhalers to change their eating behaviours. Put your fork or spoon down between each mouthful if that will help. Engage in conversation if you are eating with others. Or think of your own technique to slow yourself down if you rush your food. You need to pay attention when you eat to *how* you eat.

Watch Portion Size

Now, back to the stomach, the first place food lands after you swallow it. Make a fist and observe its size. That is how big your stomach is without any food in it. Tiny, isn't it? So, think about what happens when you pile your plate high in the evening and swallow that big mountain of food. Your stomach has to stretch to accommodate it. And food sits in the stomach for a minimum of 30 minutes to allow the stomach acid and other digestive juices to begin to break down the food.

Once your stomach gets used to being stretched, it expects it every day, and this stretching is the reason why, if you decide to eat less or go on a "diet", you tend to feel hungry after your meals for around four days, as it can take a few days for the nerve endings around your stomach pouch to shrink back. The nerves fire when they reach a certain stretching point and send a message to the brain to let you know you have eaten.

This is one of the numerous mechanisms we have that has the potential to tell us to stop eating, that we have had enough. Trouble is, for some the stomach is so used to being stretched that, by the time the nerves fire, we may have already over-eaten, started to feel lousy, and begun to berate ourselves.

The process described above is how carbohydrates let us know we have eaten. With fat and protein, however, as soon as we start to chew, messages are already being sent from the mouth to the satiety centre of the brain to let us know we are eating. These signals usually reach the brain within five minutes of chewing, while the stomach-stretch method can take more like 20 minutes. This explains why it is important to include fats and/or protein with each meal, as you are likely to eat less and be satisfied with less total food for that meal than if you simply ate carbohydrates on their own.

A rough guide to the amount of food we need to eat at each meal is approximately two fist-sized servings of concentrated food, such as proteins or carbohydrates. You can, and need, to add as many greens (non-starch vegetables and/or salad) to that as you like. Although greens have a high nutrient content, they are mostly water, as we discussed in the Beautiful Hydration chapter. Remember that.

Wake Up Your Stomach Acid pH

Food arrives at the stomach after you chew and swallow it. The aroma of food, as well as the chewing action itself, stimulates stomach acid production, which is an exceptionally important substance when it comes to great digestion. Stomach acid's role is to break food down. Imagine your food is a big, long string of circles as shown in the first row below. It is the job of the stomach acid to go chop, chop, chop, and break the circles apart into smaller bunches, as the second row illustrates.

OOOOOOOOOOOOOOOOOOOOOOOOO
⇓ (stomach acid)
OOO   OO OOO   OOO   OO   OOOO   OO

Digestion: The action of stomach acid on whole foods breaks them down into their smaller components.

There are specific, ideal pH ranges for each tissue and fluid in the body. In scientific terms, pH refers to the concentration of hydrogen ions present, but you don't need to worry about that to understand this very important process.

To recap, pH is a measure of acidity or alkalinity. Its range is based on a scale of 1 to 14, with 1 being the acid end of the spectrum and 14 being the alkaline end; 7 is neutral. Every fluid, every tissue, every cell of your body has a pH at which it performs optimally. The optimal pH of stomach acid is around 1.9, which is so acidic it would burn you if it touched your skin. But it doesn't burn you while it is nicely housed inside your stomach, as the cells that line the stomach itself not only produce stomach acid but are also designed to withstand the super-acidic conditions.

For many of us, though, the pH of our stomach acid is not acidic enough, and it may have a pH far greater than 1.9, which is not ideal for digestion. To be precise, animal proteins are optimally digested at a pH of 1.9, while starch is optimally digested at a pH of 2.1 which may not seem like much number-wise, but inside your body for some (not everyone) it can mean the difference between a flat abdomen and a bloated abdomen after a meal. A professor in the United States has been researching the pH of stomach acid in various groups of people who have been diagnosed with specific conditions, such as children with autism spectrum disorder (ASD). Many children with ASD have been found to have a stomach acid pH of around four, far too high to effectively digest protein or starch.

Adults with reflux or indigestion tend to assume that the burning sensation they experience with heartburn means they are producing too much acid when the opposite is usually true. They are usually not making enough stomach acid and/or the pH of it is too high. To understand this, remember the food-as-a-string-of-circles analogy and that stomach acid plays a vital role in breaking the circles apart. A pH that is much higher than 1.9 cannot effectively break the circles apart, and larger segments of, for example, seven circles in length may be the result. The body knows that if something seven circles in length continues along the digestive tract, it is not going to be able to further digest these partially broken-down circles. Rather than allowing that food to proceed down into the small intestine for the next part of its journey, the body regurgitates the food in an attempt to get rid of it, and you then experience the acid burn. It "burns" you, because anything with a pH that is too acidic for the tissue to which it is exposed will create a burning sensation. When the acid is contained inside the stomach pouch, all is well; however, when it escapes out of this area, the lining of the oesophagus and the first part of the small intestine are not designed to cope with such acidic contents. Many people with reflux respond well to the stimulation of stomach acid and/or omitting problematic foods, and experience much fewer symptoms as a result.

As mentioned, stomach acid is stimulated by chewing and the aroma of food, as well as by the consumption of lemon juice and apple cider vinegar (ACV). The chewing action sends a message to the brain to send a message to the stomach to let it know that food is on its way. When we inhale our food, this doesn't happen. Historically, we took much longer to prepare our meals, and the slow-cooking processes generated an aroma of the upcoming meal, signalling the stomach that food was on its way. Lemon juice and ACV physically stimulate the production of stomach acid. If you haven't consumed either of these before, it is best to initially dilute them and ideally consume them 5 to 20 minutes before breakfast (or all of your main meals if that appeals). For example, you might begin with half a teaspoon of ACV in as much water as you like. Over the coming days and weeks, you could gradually work up to having one tablespoon of ACV while you gradually decrease the amount of water. If you prefer lemon juice, start with the juice of half a lemon diluted to your tastes with *warm* water, and gradually work up to having the juice of a whole lemon in less warm water. If you use lemon, it can be a good idea to brush your teeth after your meals to prevent any potential problems with tooth enamel in the future. Use these tips to wake your stomach acid up before you eat!

The Potential Effect of Drinking Water with Meals

We need the pH of our stomach acid to sit at around 1.9. Water has a pH of 7 (neutral pH), or above, depending on the mineral content (the higher the mineral content, the higher/more alkaline the pH). When you add a liquid with a pH of 7 or more to one with a pH of 1.9, what do you potentially do to the stomach acid? You dilute it. And we need all of the digestive fire we can muster to get the maximum nourishment out of our food and the best out of us. In my ideal world, we wouldn't drink water for 30 minutes on either side of eating.

You do not need to be concerned about the water content of food, nor do you need to focus on omitting all beverages at every meal. Simply aim to drink water between meals, not with meals! It can be a challenging habit to break. Set yourself a goal of not drinking with meals for one week … and then preferably keep the new habit going. Or add a squeeze of fresh lemon juice if you want water with your meal. Just cut it out for a week, one little week out of your very long life, and see if you feel any different.

Stimulate the pH Gradient of the Digestive System

Once food has been somewhat broken down in the stomach, it moves through the pyloric sphincter, a one-way valve leading into the duodenum, which is the beginning of the small intestine. In your body this valve is located in the middle, or just slightly on the left, of the chest, just below the bra line.

While food is in the stomach, messages are sent to the pancreas to secrete sodium bicarbonate, which has a highly alkaline pH, along with digestive enzymes. The bicarbonate is designed to protect the lining of the first part of the small intestine, as well as to allow digestion to continue. What is known as a "pH gradient" is established all the way along the digestive tract, and each region of the big long tube has an ideal pH. When the pH gradient is not established in the stomach — that is, when the pH is higher than ideal — digestion problems are likely further along the tract. These may be symptoms of the small or large intestine, such as bloating, pain, or excessive wind. The absorption of nutrients may also be compromised. Insufficient pancreatic bicarbonate production may also cause digestive symptoms, such as a burning sensation underneath the stomach in the valve area described above. Pain in this area can also indicate that the gallbladder needs some support or investigation. It is best to consult with your health professional about this if you feel discomfort in this area.

The best way to let the pancreas know that it needs to jump to action and produce bicarbonate and digestive enzymes is to have good stomach acid production at optimal pH. The digestive system runs off a cascade of signals from one organ or area to the next, via the brain. Use the suggested strategies, especially chewing food well, to stimulate the pancreas to fulfil its role.

There are occasions when I have suggested clients use supplements of pancreatic enzymes, and this is appropriate if there is a genuine lack of digestive enzymes rather than simply poor stomach acid conditions. I usually suggest the aforementioned strategies before trialling supplements; however, when symptoms are severe and once other causes have been ruled out, a gastroenterologist may measure pancreatic enzyme levels.

Promote Absorption

As food moves through the small bowel, digestive enzymes are secreted from the pancreas and the brush border (lining) of the small intestine. The role of these enzymes is to continue what the stomach acid began, which is to continue to break down the food we have eaten into its smallest, most basic components. It is in the small intestine where you absorb all of the goodness (vitamins and minerals) out of your food. Think about that. All of the nutrients that keep you alive are drawn out of your food and move across into your blood so that your body can use those nutrients to do all of the life-sustaining jobs they do. The small intestine is where the nutrients in your food move from the tube that is your digestive tract into the blood, which is obviously a different set of tubes. This is how we are nourished, and it is how you stay alive!

Alcohol and vitamin B_{12} are virtually the only substances you absorb directly out of your stomach, rather than via your small intestine, and into your blood. Alcohol tends to be in your blood within five minutes of consuming it, which is why humans may get tipsy if they drink on an empty stomach.

Just because you eat something, though, doesn't mean you get all of the goodness out of it. If a food, for example, contains 10 milligrams of zinc, you don't necessarily absorb the whole 10 milligrams when you eat it. The absorption of nutrients is dependent on a whole host of factors, some of which have been discussed above. If you inhale your food, drink water with your meals, or have poor stomach acid production, for example, you may absorb very little of the goodness in your food. Nutrients are essential for life, and the *way* you are eating — let alone the foods you might be choosing — may be robbing you of some of the goodness your food provides, which can have an impact on both inner health and outer beauty. Give yourself the best opportunity to absorb as much goodness out of your food as possible through applying the tips above. It may add energy to your years and years to your life.

Address Niggling Pain

Many clients describe an on-again, off-again pain that hits them quite low down on the right-hand side of their abdomen. If you place your little finger on your right hip bone and use your thumb to find your navel, this pain tends to be located about halfway in between on that diagonal line. This is the ileocaecal valve, where the small intestine meets the large intestine. Many people have mistaken ileocaecal valve pain for appendicitis, as the appendix is located not far from this area. Always see a medical professional to diagnose your pain.

For many, pain begins in this area after food poisoning or a stomach bug (infection), after travelling, usually overseas, or camping. When you had the bug, you might have had bouts of diarrhoea. Even though the obvious symptoms of the causative infection have long since gone, it is as though the nasty little critters that caused the original upset tummy have taken up residence in the valve. Or perhaps they have changed its function. To remedy this pain, there are numerous options to try. One is to release the reflex connected to this valve by rubbing the area with your fingertips 20 times in an anticlockwise circular motion with reasonable pressure, not so it hurts you but also not with super-soft fingers. Another option is to use antiparasitic herbs, such as Chinese wormwood and black walnut, every day for four to eight weeks, before each main meal. The other potential remedy is one of my favourite substances on Earth: Lugol's iodine. The liquid of potassium iodide is not only a source of iodine, necessary for so many body functions, but it acts as a potent anti-parasitic agent that seems to help clear the last of the nasty critters from this important valve. It is possible to overdose on iodine, so it is best to check your dosage with a health professional to make sure the dose is right for you.

Promote Good Gut Bacteria

Once the food gets to the large intestine, can you guess what lives there? Bacteria. On average, an adult will have three to four kilograms of bacteria living in their colon. So, just as an aside, every time you weigh yourself remember that three to four of the kilos you see in that number on the scales is made up of gut bacteria that are essential for life; another reason why it is crazy that we weigh ourselves.

Some of the bacteria in your large bowel (colon) are good guys and some are bad guys. You want more good guys than bad guys. The role of the gut bacteria is to ferment whatever you give them. To come back to the circle concept of food illustrated previously, gut bugs love it when you give them something that is one or even two circles in size. They know what to do with that. But if a previous digestive process was not completed sufficiently, the gut bacteria in our colon may be presented with fragments of food that are five or even seven circles in size, and all they know to do with any food is ferment it.

What word springs to mind when you think of fermentation? I love asking this question at my seminars, as the answers usually amuse me as well as the audience. People will often say "beer", "wine", "sauerkraut"! But usually I eventually get the answer I am after, which is gas. Fermentation involves bacterial action on a food source, and the subsequent production of gas. Some gases are essential to the health of the cells that line our gut, while others seem to irritate the gut and give us a bloated, uncomfortable stomach as the day progresses, whether we have eaten in a healthy way or not.

The trouble with a bloated stomach for many women is that it messes with their brain. When they look down and see a swollen tummy, something inside immediately communicates to every cell of their body that they are fat, whether they consciously think this thought or not. Many of my clients go up a size around the waist as the day progresses even though they feel they have eaten with their health in mind. This can add a layer of stress to a woman's life that they just don't need or understand. It is especially stressful because they can't fathom why it is happening. Sometimes it is the foods you are choosing. Sometimes it is the bugs that live in your colon.

Sometimes it is because of poor digestion further up the process, such as insufficient stomach acid. In traditional Chinese medicine (TCM), bloating is often considered a spleen and/or liver picture, and a TCM practitioner is likely to use acupuncture and/or herbs to support the spleen and liver. Sometimes bloating is due to too much coffee or from stress and living in the red zone (adrenalin).

Address Stress

Poor digestion can be due to stress or, more precisely, adrenalin. As we have discussed elsewhere, stress causes the adrenalin to divert the blood supply away from your digestive processes and concentrate the blood in your periphery, your arms and legs. With the blood not focused on digestion, you are more likely to get out of the perceived danger you are in, and it keeps you focused on escaping the danger. If blood were still concentrated on the digestive system, there is a risk you would be distracted by food, putting your survival at risk. These concepts have been explored in detail in the Not-So-Beautiful Stress Hormones chapter.

Ensure Complete Bowel Evacuation

In dealing with clients one-on-one, I have had to work out ways to extract information from people using words that accurately investigate what is going on for that person. Many years ago, one of the questions I originally found difficult to phrase was around how empty someone felt after they had used their bowels. I tried to dream up ways to word this question so that it wouldn't make clients feel uncomfortable, but also so that I could gain more insight into how their bowel was functioning. As with most things, a client turned out to have the answer. While asking him about his bowel habits, he said, "You know what? My greatest discomfort comes from incomplete evacuation." There they were. The words I needed. So, early on in my consultation work with people, I started asking about feelings of incomplete evacuation. For some, it is not an issue at all. They have no idea what I am talking about when I mention it. For others, they are so excited that someone has finally given them the words to describe such frustrating discomfort. They wouldn't answer yes if I asked them if they were constipated, as they may use their bowels every day. It is just that when they do go to the toilet, they feel like there is more to come but it doesn't eventuate and evacuate.

This feeling can be the result of numerous scenarios. It may be insufficient digestive processes as outlined previously. It may be inadequate production of digestive enzymes due to poor signalling, or a damaged or inflamed brush border. It may be a food allergy or intolerance. It could be related to fibre or dehydration. It can be stress hormones causing the muscles surrounding the bowel to contract and hold onto waste. It may be a magnesium deficiency not allowing the walls of the bowel to relax and allow the thorough passage of waste. Or the thyroid gland may not be working optimally. TCM teaches us that it is insufficient spleen and/or liver energy. The list of scenarios is almost endless. Digestion support strategies are also covered on the blog at: www.drlibby.com/bioresources

Dietary Change: Dietary Trials

One option to improve this challenge is to have a health professional help you get to the bottom of it and remedy the situation. You might increase your green vegetable intake and decrease the processed foods in your diet for a week and see if that makes a difference, especially given that green vegetables are good sources of magnesium, water and fibre, amongst other things. You may be suspicious of a food or a group of foods that are causing this feeling for you, but because you love this food you are reluctant to remove it. I cannot encourage you enough to remove your suspicious food from your diet for a *trial* period of two weeks (four is even better). Two little weeks out of your very long life — an expression I use regularly with clients to highlight the relatively short time period necessary to potentially offer enormous insight into their health challenges. For some, however, a longer trial of three months is necessary. You may get an answer to your challenge over the trial period and, if not, you can relax and thoroughly enjoy this food without silently worrying. But I can hear you already asking: "What if it works? What does that mean? Will I never eat that food again?" My answer is always that it is your choice.

I have witnessed people be resistant to dietary change, but after a time feel so different, so much better, that they have no desire to ever go back to the way they used to eat. I have met others who, even though they may feel better, may still miss a food terribly. If it is the latter scenario, I suggest to them after the trial that it is a good thing that now they know. It is no longer a mystery to them why they feel this way. Then they are in control. Unless the problem is a true allergy, I find that when people are strong — meaning when they are very robust from a digestion perspective — their gut will tolerate this food better than if they are stressed. Either way, once you know, you are in control, and it is your choice. You know that if you have an important event coming up, you might like to avoid the culprit food for a time so you feel and look your best for your occasion. Again, unless the food is a true allergy for you, your tolerance of it may change and improve over time, especially with a focus on gut healing and stress management. Don't think that because it hurts you today it always will. Your body changes and renews itself constantly. Just know there is a reason for your symptom. It is simply a matter of finding your answer.

Softening Waste

One of the reasons I am so concerned with bowel evacuation is that, if this process is inefficient, waste can remain inside the bowel for too long. While it is there, it is fermenting. This can give the liver additional and unnecessary toxins to process, as well as "suffocating" the cells that line the colon. The waste can also dry out and harden, sticking itself to the lining of the bowel wall, narrowing the tube through which the new waste can flow. If you have ever seen soil in the middle of a drought, cracked, dried-out, and unable to absorb a brief shower of rain, that is the way hardened faeces can behave in your colon.

If this scenario occurs, waste can only move through the middle of this newly formed, faeces-lined tube, and the efficiency of waste elimination is decreased. The old, hard, compacted faecal matter remains. When the cells that line the bowel are coated with hard faeces, they are unable to "breathe", and a process that was once described in medical textbooks as autointoxication can ensue. To remedy this, chamomile is one of the best things you can take. Either drink lots of tea, or take capsules with each meal. Once the waste has dried out, it is difficult to rehydrate it so it can move through and be excreted. Chamomile softens the waste and helps the bowel wall relax.

Colonics

Another potential remedy is one about which many people have very strong opinions: colon hydrotherapy, or colonics. This process involves a tube being inserted into a person's rectum through which warm or cool water gently flows. This allows the hardened faecal matter to soften, like heavy, consistent rain on dried-out soil, allowing the large bowel to empty fully, often getting rid of built-up waste that may have been there for a very long time. I have had clients tell me that the waste they excreted during their first colonic was black, inferring that it may have been there for many years, interfering with healthy bowel function. I had a lady once tell me she saw popcorn in the viewing pipe during her colonic and she knows that the last time she ate popcorn was at the movies over six months ago!

Colonics polarize people. The idea either appeals to you or it doesn't. There is no middle ground with people's love or dislike of colon hydrotherapy. I encourage you, though, not to lose sight of the effect that trends have had on medicine. Up until the early 1900s, colonics were accepted as part of general medicine. Doctors understood the importance of good bowel evacuation, and considered colonics to be a normal treatment method for a host of health conditions, not just bowel issues. Coffee enemas were actually cited in the *Merck Manual for Doctors* for liver detoxification until 1972.

With a well-functioning bowel, an enormous load is taken off not only the digestive system but also the liver, one of the organs primarily responsible for cleaning our body. Help prevent bowel cancer by ensuring efficient bowel evacuation using methods that suit you! Always seek advice from a health professional before undertaking colon hydrotherapy if it appeals to you.

Gut Integrity and Opioid Effects

An additional concept within digestive health is not only fascinating but has wide-ranging effects on how we feel and function, including gut transit time (how quickly food moves through the digestive system), mood, concentration, and, potentially, food addictions. This concept is known as the opioid excess theory.

The cells that line a healthy small intestine look like a row of neatly stacked bricks with finger-like projections (called villi), side-by-side as demonstrated in the picture below.

vitamin c

⎽⎽⎽⎽⎽⎽⎽⎽⎽⎽⎽⎽⎽⎽⎽⎽⎽⎽

◡◡◡◡◡◡◡◡◡◡◡◡◡◡◡◡◡

0000 →

⋂⋂⋂⋂⋂⋂⋂⋂⋂⋂⋂⋂⋂⋂⋂⋂⋂

⎽⎽⎽⎽⎽⎽⎽⎽⎽⎽⎽⎽⎽⎽⎽⎽⎽⎽

zinc

A healthy gut: Food (circles) travelling through a healthy mature intestine move straight ahead. Only nutrients (for example, Vitamin C and zinc) enter the blood vessels that closely follow the intestines.

In a healthy gut, only the tiny nutrients (vitamins and minerals) diffuse (move) through the gut wall into the blood, and this is the precious process through which we are nourished and stay alive. However, the cells that line the gut can come apart, as if the bricks have gaps between them, illustrated below. This is, in fact, how our gut is when we are born.

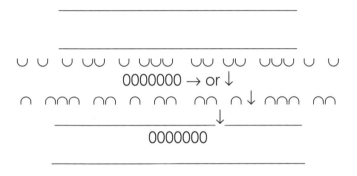

A "leaky" gut: Food (circles) travel through an immature gut or a "leaky" intestine. Microscopic, poorly digested fragments of food can escape out of the gut and enter the blood.

When we are born, the cells that line our digestive system are a distance apart, which is why we can't feed all foods to newborns; foods must be gradually introduced to a child over time to prevent allergic reactions as the gut matures. The gut is immature when we are born, and it slowly matures from birth until reaching full maturity somewhere between the ages of two and five, depending on the individual child and their health and life experiences in the early years. Sadly, for some this maturation process may be stunted by constant ill health until gut health is addressed.

The cells that line the gut can, however, also come apart during adulthood as a result of a gastrointestinal infection or stress. The chronic production of stress hormones can compromise the integrity of the gut cells and signal to them that they need to move further apart so that more nutrition can get through to the blood, as nutrient requirements increase during times of stress. Everything about us is geared for survival.

When food travels through a gut with good cell-lining integrity, it can only go straight ahead. However, if it travels through a gut in which the cells have come apart, it may go straight ahead or it may move out of the gut and into the blood. Fragments of food are not intended to enter the blood. Nutrients, the vitamins and minerals from food, are. If fragments of food enter the bloodstream, the immune system, which is what protects you from infection, thinks that the food fragment is a germ and it mounts an immune response against it. This is one way adults develop food sensitivities. Poor gut integrity is also described as "leaky gut". Once you were able to eat anything without a problem, and now certain foods seem to cause you grief. This process can be healed by minimizing the irritation to the gut lining, which can mean avoiding some foods or ingredients for a period of time, while also working on the gut integrity. Aloe vera juice to start the day can also assist an irritated gut.

Often people are able to tolerate the foods that cause them grief once we have worked out why they have the leaky gut symptoms in the first place. Did the problem begin as a result of stress or an infection? The power to heal the symptoms is always in the "why".

The blood supply into which the food fragments flow is the same blood supply that goes to your brain. Humans have what is known as the blood–brain barrier, a semi-permeable layer separating the peripheral blood supply from that of the brain. The blood–brain barrier was always considered to be a highly selective membrane that only allowed substances into the brain that would be of benefit. However, research has now shown us that this is not the case. In cases where gut permeability is increased, the blood–brain barrier is often suspected of having the same increased permeability.

If we could literally see the food fragments, their structure is very similar to that of opioids. Opioids are substances that help humans feel good. They also modulate pain. We have our own natural feel-good hormones, endorphins, which have an opioid-based structure. In our brain and in our gut, we have what are called opioid receptors. To review: just because your body makes a substance (chemical messenger/hormone) that doesn't mean you necessarily get the effects of that substance. For you to get the effect generated by that hormone, the substance must bind to a receptor, just like a lock and a key fitting together. In this case, when we make endorphins and they bind to the opioid receptors, we feel pleasure. Heroine and morphine are opioids, and they, too, bind to the opioid receptors in the brain. Anything that gives a human pleasure has the potential to be addictive, hence the aforementioned drugs. You can also see from this example how someone might become addicted to exercise. Activity certainly generates endorphins when we partake. So whatever give you pleasure — like a sunset, a spin class, a football game, or a child's laughter — what has happened in that moment is that you have made endorphins and they have bound to opioid receptors, and you have felt pleasure.

How does this relate to food and beauty? Some of the fragments of food that can escape out of a leaky gut into the bloodstream can also have an opioid structure. These include beta-casomorphine and gluteomorphine. They are partially digested fragments of casein (the major protein in cow's milk products) and gluten (the major protein in wheat, rye, barley, oats, and triticale). Just like endorphins, these opioids from food also have the capacity to bind to the opioid receptors in the brain and very subtly make us feel good. The effect is not usually noticed as an enormous boost in mood, but the person will often feel as though they can't live without this food, and they will feel as though they *have* to eat it in some form daily or even at every meal.

I have seen this to be the case with countless clients. If a patient has a set of symptoms that warrants them omitting a food from their diet for a trial period to see if it will make a difference, some people have no problem. There is no resistance. Others will beg me not to take them off a food for a trial, yet they are seeing me because they want results, and all I am asking is four measly weeks of omitting a particular food that may just give them the answer to some of their health concerns! I am not judging someone who responds in this way; I am simply pointing out to you that the power food can have over an individual can be just like an addiction. An individual's connection to a certain food is often highly emotional, and also potentially physical, through this opioid mechanism.

Food was never intended to fill these roles for humans. However, on a physical level, where there is a leaky gut, it is possible that the opioid effect that some foods have the potential to create might be one of the factors behind food addictions and, hence, for some, over-eating or eating and not feeling like you can stop. This is an area that deserves much more research, time, and money, as the opioid excess theory may be involved in numerous health conditions as well as obesity. Much research has already been done in relation to children with autism and adults with schizophrenia, where these exorphins (opioids from an exogenous source — that is, consumed rather than made by the body) have been found to play a role in the expression of symptoms of these conditions.

Food not only has the capacity to affect our skin, body shape, and size, but also our mood. Our digestion of some foods may also be incomplete, leading to the generation of an opioid effect and addiction to particular foods. If you suspect this process is going on for you, omit all sources of that dietary component (gluten and/or casein) for a trial period of four weeks. The first four to seven days will be the most difficult, but persevere. The results may be enormously worth it. If you do omit significant dietary components from your diet for extended periods, it can be useful to consult a health professional to make sure you do not miss out on any nutrients essential for your health.

Support the Spleen — the TCM Perspective

The spleen rules digestion in traditional Chinese medicine (TCM). In TCM, each organ is considered to have its own vital energy, as well as there being whole-body energy. If spleen energy is down, you will feel your usual hunger for meals, but as soon as you eat even a small amount, you will feel full and possibly bloated. Your short-term memory is likely to not be what it once was, and you may possibly feel like you eat like a bird yet your weight continues to escalate. You can eat and exercise with a real commitment, but if spleen energy is low, from a TCM perspective, you won't feel like your best self.

Stimulating spleen energy can make a real difference. Acupuncture will do this, as will bitter herbs. Spleen energy will go low in the first place from what is simply described as overthinking. The busy mind, relentlessly thinking of the next thing you need to do, takes energy away from the vital process of digestion every day, according to TCM principles. The spleen may also lose some of its strength if liver or kidney (adrenals sit on top of the kidneys) energy is overbearing or low. Working with a wonderful TCM practitioner can also help you heal your gut, which in turn helps every aspect of your well-being, including your skin.

Consider Food Combining

Food combining can be a wonderful approach to eating that can enhance digestion, energy, vitality, and fat loss, and it can be a great way to combat a bloated tummy. It involves a few simple principles, including eating animal protein separate from starchy carbohydrates. In practice, that means no meat and potatoes on the same plate. It means that if you eat meat, chicken, or fish, you eat it with high-water vegetables and no starchy vegetables, such as potato, sweet potato, pumpkin, corn, or any other starchy foods, such as pasta, bread, or rice. If you eat vegetable protein, such as one of the many types of lentils, chickpeas, or beans, then, using the food combining principles, you do not eat meat with these foods, but instead any vegetable at all, including starchy ones if they appeal. If you feel like eating rice, then, with food combining, it needs to be a vegetarian meal. Oils and other foods rich in fats, including avocado, can be eaten with either animal-based meals or starch-based meals.

Another principle of food combining is that fruit is only consumed as your first meal and not again during the day, due to some people's digestive inefficiencies to metabolize fructose. For some, instead of digesting it, it ferments, which can lead to a range of gut symptoms. You are also encouraged to omit all refined sugar and processed foods, as the main goal of food combining is to support your blood chemistry in remaining effortlessly alkaline.

I know people who live by the concept of food

combining and feel spectacular. For others, for whom this seems extreme, but who still want to try it, I suggest they apply the zigzag principle. This means that most of the time they follow food combining principles (zig), while one day a week, or two to three meals a week, they relax the principles and they zag. This approach is more sustainable for some; you are still able to dine out and enjoy all foods, whatever combination arrives on your plate, but just not every day. Remember, it is what you do every day that impacts on your health, not what you do sometimes. It is important to note that this latter statement is *not* applicable to true food allergies — they must strictly omitted from the diet.

Food combining is a structured way of eating that allows some individuals to thrive. I have seen this approach to diet truly change people's lives. For others, eating this way might take every aspect of joy out of their life. If this is the case for you, then focusing on food combining is not for you right now, or perhaps the zigzag concept might appeal. I am certainly not prescribing this for you. I simply want to offer you options to help you experience your best health and sparkle.

REMEMBER ...

Digestion is central and essential to every process in our body, which is why, when supporting both inner health and outer beauty, it is the base from which we build. As around 80 per cent of your immune system lines your gut, when gut function is impaired it can have a significant impact on the immune system, with some researchers suggesting that this is where some autoimmune conditions originate.

So, whether your focus is optimizing your health and well-being, and/or improving a challenging or diseased gut, body fat management, or resolving congested skin, understanding your digestive system is a crucial step in your *Beauty from the Inside Out* approach.

Remember the following important tips:

- Slow down! Chew your food. Swallow each mouthful before you put the next mouthful in.

- Include fats and/or protein with each meal, as you are likely to eat less and be satisfied with less total food for that meal than if you simply eat carbohydrates on their own.

- Wake up your stomach acid before you eat, by using lemon juice in warm water or apple cider vinegar before meals, breakfast in particular.

- Drink water between meals, not with meals.

- Use the strategies throughout *Beauty from the Inside Out* to ensure efficient bowel evacuation, such as good hydration, magnesium, liver support herbs.

- Omit a food you feel you cannot live without for a trial period of four weeks. The first four to seven days will be the most difficult, but persevere. The results may be enormously worth it.

- Working with a practitioner of traditional Chinese medicine can also help you heal your gut.

- Try aloe vera juice to start your day if you have a particularly irritated gut.

- Eat in a calm state.

- Look at your food while you eat it. Do not read or watch television while you eat.

- If you suspect a parasite infection, the herbs black walnut and Chinese wormwood are excellent, as is oregano oil.

- If you suspect you have some not-so-nice gut bacteria that are fermenting your food, apply all of these strategies first to see if that helps, as often the bad guys have been able to take over because of the pH of the large intestine, and this is mostly influenced by what goes on higher up the in the digestive system. If these strategies don't work, trial a probiotic supplement that is based on *Bifidobacterium* species.

- If you suspect you are reacting to a food, strictly omit that food from your diet for a period of four weeks. If it makes no difference, bring it back. If it helps, leave it out for three months, and then try it again. Or, if you are happy to go without it, then do so. If it is a food that is a rich source of nutrients — for example, gluten-containing foods tend to be a good source of B vitamins — then you will need to supplement. It will also be necessary to supplement with a mineral supplement that contains a combination of calcium, magnesium, manganese, boron, and vitamin D if you omit dairy products. This is of lesser importance if your diet is caffeine-free, plant-based, and highly alkaline. It is best to seek the guidance of a health professional if you are going to omit food(s) to get a resolution of your symptoms on a longer-term basis.

- Chamomile is one of the best remedies for constipation and complete evacuation. This is because it can soften the waste and help the bowel wall relax. Either drink lots of tea, or take capsules with each meal. I am a huge fan of this beautiful herb.

- Trial food combining principles if that appeals to you and you feel like you have tried everything else to solve gut dysfunction.

- Base your diet on real food, not processed food; your body knows how to digest real food.

When you arise in the morning, think of what a precious privilege it is to be alive: to breathe, to think, to enjoy, to love.

Marcus Aurelius

Chapter 7
Beautiful Sleep:
the foundation of beauty

Sleep is a topic I feel incredibly passionate about for a huge number of reasons. When we are exhausted, everything in life feels more difficult. So I want to give you very practical information, things you can actually apply to your life to make a really big difference in this area. Before we discuss what to do about sleep that is not restorative, it is first important for you to understand *why* sleep can become disrupted and ineffective in its purpose of rest, repair, and restoration. I also want to show you how common it is now to sleep poorly — common, but not normal, as I like to say.

In February 2013, my team and I conducted a survey asking people who read our Facebook page (facebook.com/DrLibbyLive) about their sleep. Over 500 people answered our questions. Of those, 97 per cent shared with us that they wake up tired.

Only three per cent of people reported waking up with energy.[3] Think about that. Waking unrefreshed is a really big deal. Furthermore, the majority of people who responded couldn't sleep through the night either, and this is an area that, once it is optimal, will make a significant difference to so many aspects of your health and beauty. As I said, everything feels more difficult when we are exhausted. So let's get you sleeping restoratively.

Sleep, and the rest and repair it offers our body, is critical to life. With great sleep, we have improved memory, cognition, and better immune function. Sometimes when I talk about immune function, I sense that the importance of this system doesn't fully register with some people. Many people simply link great immune function with minimizing how many colds and flus they get. Yet your immune function is critical in the prevention of cancer, as well as in the prevention of autoimmune diseases, such as multiple sclerosis, lupus, and coeliac disease, all of which are on the rise. Taking great care of our immune system is of immense importance to our long-term health and quality of life, and sleep plays an enormous role in whether our immune system is able to function appropriately or not.

With restorative sleep, we have improved mood, enhanced physical and emotional resilience, increased

---

3   Please note that this is not scientific research, but a survey. One could argue that people who are drawn to learn more about their body and/or who have challenges with sleep may be more likely to comment on a sleep survey. I am simply pointing out that large numbers of people don't sleep restoratively.

physical endurance, and better hormonal function. When our sleep cycles are disrupted, both our stress hormones and our sex hormone balances can be impacted, as you now understand from previous chapters.

Everything works better with restorative sleep: our digestive system, our sex hormone balance, our mood, our skin, and even our thyroid function. A recent clinical trial found that sleep quality impacts skin function and aging. If you have poor sleep quality or do not get enough sleep, your skin finds it harder to recover from free radical damage, such as sun exposure and environmental toxins.

I wanted to open this chapter by showing you just how far-reaching amazing sleep can be, because you may just think "Oh, I wake up tired most of the time, but isn't that normal?" No, it is common, but it is *not* normal. Many people blame age for why they start to feel more and more tired as the years go by, but it doesn't have to be this way. If low energy truly was down to age, then every 82-year-old I know would be exhausted, and they're not! We can make a really big difference to how we feel and function, both on the inside and the outside, through good-quality sleep.

SLEEP REQUIRED

How much sleep do you actually need? Our requirements vary based on our gender, our age, and our physical demands. There are studies that suggest that adults have a very basic sleep requirement of seven to eight hours per night. Other compelling studies show eight to eight and a half hours per night is actually critical for all of the vital repair work that has to go on inside your body while you are asleep.

We are essentially the health of our cells, and cellular repair takes place during sleep. Everything from skin cells to the cells that make up our muscles need repair work overnight. When cells are working optimally, we look and feel our best. I want to remind you that we cannot fight our biology: our biology is our biology, and we need eight hours of sleep a night. When we are not getting that, all sorts of bodily functions can be disrupted. So, let's help you achieve blissful sleep!

Sleep requirements tend to be based somewhat on our age. Newborn babies need a lot of sleep; although many of you may have experienced first-hand that some babies need more than others. Some like or need a lot of sleep, perhaps 18 hours a day, and then there are those who need somewhat less, perhaps 12 or 14 hours a day. Infants, toddlers, and preschoolers need less sleep than newborns, but still substantially more than teenagers. Sleep needs continue to gradually decline, and by the time children are teenagers they need between about eight and a half and nine and a quarter hours per night. I have deep concerns, however, over what's happening for our teenagers, because many of them are taking backlit devices to bed, such as iPads, laptops, and cell phones. And the light that is omitted from these devices can significantly disrupt the production of the sleep hormone called melatonin. Light destroys melatonin, as you will learn more about in a moment, which is one reason why I have deep concerns for teens who may not be getting enough hours of sleep to do the vital growth and repair work that needs to happen. As mentioned above, an adult's biological requirement for sleep is essentially seven to nine hours of sleep per night.

If you have been jotting down things that speak to you as you have gone through this book, now is a particularly important time to keep that paper close. Your willingness to open and consider new choices in all the areas we have discussed so far begins with a good night's sleep.

SLEEP ATTAINED

While I was gathering research for an online sleep seminar I created as well as for this book, I was curious about how much sleep people are truly getting, particularly because sleep is often referred to as "beauty sleep".

The data in the following graph shows sleep patterns for people in New Zealand from 1960 until 2002.

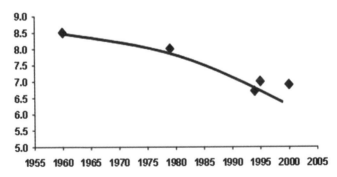

Self-reported number of hours of sleep per night: Note that the decline is a concern (Source: Medscape)

In New Zealand in 1960, people reported that they

were getting about eight and half hours of sleep each night. By 2002, the number of hours per night had dropped to six and a half. If the graph continued on its current trajectory, you can see that by now, 2013, we'd be down to more like six hours a night, or even five and a half hours per night, which is of grave concern to our health, our longevity, how we feel, how we function, and how we appear every single day. Too many people aren't getting enough sleep. I also appreciate that many people make an enormous effort to get plenty of sleep but their body won't cooperate and let them sleep.

When I was the programme manager at the beautiful Gwinganna Lifestyle Retreat in Australia, it was a joy to look after people for a week of their lives in this gorgeous setting, full of incredible natural beauty. For those at the retreat, all meals were taken care of; the meals themselves were beautiful and also nourishing. Participants didn't have laundry to take care of or groceries to buy. Lush rooms, lovely spa treatments, and access to restorative movement ... The entire week was all about each individual having a transformative experience. At the end of each week, I always asked each group what they had loved the most during their stay. Countless people said that their favourite thing over the whole week was their sleep. This brought home to me just how invaluable sleep is. In the middle of a retreat, with every soul-nourishing amenity available, the best gift for so many was restorative sleep. It is amazing how we can feel when we actually sleep well and for long enough.

SLEEP AS A PRIORITY

For many people, to improve their sleep it needs to become a priority. So many people today compromise their sleep to get more done in a day. They wake up earlier and go to bed later in an attempt to get more tasks done. Yet when you deeply appreciate how non-negotiable sleep is for your health, and your beauty armoury, you make it a priority. If you find you are someone who stays up later and later in an attempt to get more things crossed off your "to-do" list, then it may take an extreme question for you to follow through with making sleep a priority. Try asking yourself: "Will anyone die if I don't get this done?" If the answer is yes, then stay up later and do it. If the answer is no, go to bed! Some of you will have to go to this extreme to make sleep a priority.

SLEEP STATS AND SLEEPING PILLS

This will help you see what a significant and widespread challenge good-quality, restorative sleep is. Many of the statistics are from New Zealand, but it is likely that the data would be relatively similar across most Western countries. Did you know:

- it takes a third of New Zealanders over 30 minutes to get to sleep?

- one complete night of sleep deprivation can be as impairing in a simulated driving test as a legally intoxicating blood-alcohol level?

- in New Zealand in 2012, almost 680,000 unique sleeping pill prescriptions were given (with a population of around 4.5 million)?

What these statistics highlight to me is that sleep is an enormous issue. It is huge for the 4.5 million people who live in New Zealand and for those throughout the Western world. With 680,000 out of approximately 4.5 million citizens using sleeping pills to fall asleep and stay asleep, this shows that a significant percentage of a representative population struggles with sleep. Some people who use sleeping tablets may use them only occasionally, or for a brief time during a particularly trying time, after a bereavement, for example, while others will use them nightly. However, the numbers are still concerning. Why has such a fundamental function of our body become such a challenge? Let's keep exploring and you will soon see why and — just as importantly — what to do about it.

A common scenario is that people go to their general practitioner (GP) and complain that they are not sleeping well. The GP, who has more and more demands placed on them, is more and more time-poor. So when a patient comes in who is not sleeping well and the patient may even ask for sleeping pills just to get things back on track, the GP might just offer the prescription And so people start, without any real investigation done into *why* they aren't sleeping well, and they take the medication, thinking they will only use it short term, just to get a good night's sleep. However, poor sleep can be just another sign the body gives you that the way you eat, drink, think, move, believe, and/or perceive needs to change.

WHAT INTERFERES WITH RESTORATIVE SLEEP?

When sleeping pills are used as a bridge, as a short-term band-aid for sleep problems, there is potentially no problem. But until the deeper issue(s) that created the sleep issue in the first place are addressed, no progress will be made that allows the person to come off the sleeping pills and begin sleeping naturally again. So people come to rely on medication for their sleep, and it is this long-term use that I am concerned about. The deeper issue(s) must be addressed or other health challenges can potentially arise. I call it "getting to the heart of the matter". And sometimes the heart of the matter is physical (biochemical), such as too much caffeine or alcohol, and sometimes it is emotional. For example, you may lie awake at night worrying that you let someone down that day.

Another great thing to ask yourself is when the last time was that you slept well. If it was when you were on holiday, you can bet that stress is playing a big role in you not sleeping well in your usual life. If the last time you slept well was in a hotel, again it may be worthwhile to consider how stress may be involved, but also look at what you are sleeping on. People often keep their beds for far too long; in a hotel, the beds tend to be newer, so it might simply be the structural support that you are getting in a hotel that allows you to rest easy. Pay attention to whether you sleep better when you have a small meal for dinner or even for some reason skip dinner. Heed the advice in the Beautiful Digestion chapter if this is the case for you, such as omitting spicy food in the evening or eating smaller portions, as this may positively impact your sleep.

Maybe the last time you slept well was after abstaining from alcohol. The reality is that alcohol disrupts rapid eye movement (REM) sleep, the fourth part of our sleep cycle, during which time the critical repair work is done inside our body. Even though alcohol actually tends to make people fall asleep quite quickly, it can disrupt our sleep cycles, as it interferes with REM sleep. Notice how alcohol affects your sleep, and consider making changes.

The last time you slept well may have been before you had children. If you sleep quite well but your sleep is interrupted because little ones need you in the night, please remember that they are young for such a short amount of time and there will come a time when they sleep through the night. Worrying about your sleep, and the disruptions that you can't do anything about, only serves to disrupt your sleep further. So I encourage you to accept that right now your sleep will be disrupted, and make the most of the nights when it is not!

Interference with Melatonin Production

Melatonin is your primary sleep hormone; it helps you fall asleep and stay asleep. Its production in your body is interfered with by light. Relatively speaking, it wasn't too long ago that we rose with the sun and rested soon after sundown. Obviously that changed with the invention of electricity.

When you expose your eyes to light too late into the evening, through any means, including the use of backlit devices, such as iPads, mobile phones, and laptops, or you work until late under bright light or watch television, it can stop your body from producing the very hormone that is necessary for great sleep. If you don't wake up refreshed, or particularly if you have trouble falling asleep, become very aware of how much light you are exposing your eyes to within two hours of bedtime. If sleep is a challenge for you, do what you can to only be in soft light in the lead-up to bedtime and make your bedroom a television- and wireless-device-free zone.

Another powerful way to help re-set your body's own natural circadian rhythm is to get up at the same time each morning and expose your eyes to light. Preferably get up and go outside and exercise. If that is not practical for you — perhaps because you have young children who need you — then, on waking, get up and fling the curtains open and notice the day and Nature outside; think of three things you are grateful for, and allow your eyes to gently be exposed to the light of this new day. Commit to doing this for a week minimum, and begin to notice the difference.

Melatonin has an antagonistic relationship with serotonin, one of our happy, calm, content hormones. Antagonistic means that both substances can't be elevated at the same time. When one is high, the other tends to be low. Your circadian rhythm guides serotonin to be high during the day, helping you to feel good, and melatonin is designed to be high through the night, supporting your sleep.

The serotonin–melatonin seesaw, as I have come to call it, is I think one of the reasons why couples tend to have big conversations in the evening. Up until late afternoon, you may have been going along just fine, content, regardless of what was or wasn't going on in your life. Your serotonin level is still OK, and you aren't focused on anything you want. Then, if serotonin levels plummet instead of gradually falling away, you may start to feel like you want something, but you don't know what it is. Whenever you ask your brain a question, it always comes up with an answer, so be very aware of the quality of questions you ask yourself! Perhaps you say, "I feel like I want something. I'm not sure what it is, but I want something. A minute ago I felt fine and now I feel like

I've got an itch I can't scratch and I want something. What do I want?!" If big things such as "I want ... to move house" or "I want ... to renovate the bathroom yesterday" or "I want ... to have a baby" don't surface, you will still be feeling like you want something, and you will decide it must be food that you want. So you will open the door of the pantry and stand there looking inside, as if the meaning of life is in that cupboard! You get what I mean.

Humans instinctively know that carbohydrate-rich foods promote serotonin production, which is partly why when the "I want something" syndrome hits you might head for the pantry. We hope that what we want is in there. Usually guilt is all we find.

The morning time can also prove to be a challenge for someone in this pattern, as serotonin can be slow to rise. As you now know, melatonin is destroyed by sunlight, which is partly why when we go outside and exercise in the morning we feel so great all day. The melatonin plummets when the retina of our eyes is exposed to light and, as a result, our serotonin surges. On a day with that hormonal profile, we can cope with anything. The flip side, though, is not so appealing. If we have gone to bed after midnight, not slept well, and have children or work to get up for, or all of these factors, we may not want to rise with the sun, as we don't feel rested. If we don't have early-morning commitments and just wander out of bed at some point during the morning, our melatonin slowly seeps away, and our serotonin slowly rises. On a day like this, we feel like we need a few coffees to get us going.

If this tale is ringing true for you, and the carb fest in the evening feels out of control, the solution is not initially dietary. Step one is to start getting up at the same time each morning and going outside and moving. Or at least open the curtains and recognize that a new day has dawned. Welcome the day with t'ai chi, a walk, or a run, whatever feels right to your body. Commit to doing this for four weeks, every day. Your sleep and your serotonin will love you for it.

Sympathetic Nervous System (SNS) Dominance

What is known as sympathetic nervous system (SNS) dominance can significantly interfere with sleep; a concept I go into great detail about in my *Rushing Woman's Syndrome* book and programmes. As you learnt earlier, the sympathetic nervous system is behind the fight-or-flight response, driven predominantly by the stress hormone adrenalin. The opposite part of the nervous system, the parasympathetic nervous system (PNS), acts as the rest, digest, repair, and reproduce arm. I could talk underwater for days about the vast impact your nervous system has on your level of well-being, but I'll keep the focus, this time, on sleep.

The challenge for so many people, and a major reason why they don't sleep well or feel and look their best, is that they are stuck in SNS dominance. I call it living from the "red zone". As you now know, historically, the only time we went into this alarm phase was when our life truly was in danger. However, today, anything that leads us to make adrenalin promotes this fight-or-flight response. And what leads us to make adrenalin? Caffeine and our perception of pressure. You'll notice that I used the word "perception" to describe pressure in the previous sentence. And that is because it is. As you read this, some of you will feel an instant frustration, and think that if I am saying that pressure is a perception then I can't possibly understand your life. But, please hear this. The reason I know that pressure is a perception is exemplified by the following scenario. Someone approaches you and rants and raves with: "You won't believe what I've got on my plate at the moment. I've got this and this and this going on and it's all going on at the same time." And depending on what your life and your perceptions are like, you may internally, or out loud, respond with: "That sounds like a walk in the park compared to what I've got going on!"

Your body doesn't understand that it is safe when you are churning out adrenalin, even if all you have done is had a few coffees and felt overwhelmed by how many emails you have! And some of you live on adrenalin and no longer even really fell stressed because you have become so used to it. It feels "normal" to you now. You tell yourself it is just how life is these days. If that resonates with you, I cannot encourage you enough to read *Rushing Woman's Syndrome*. And if you don't have time to read the book — because you are in too much of a rush — do the *Rushing Woman's Syndrome Quick Start* course (www.drlibby.com/changeyourlife) to coach yourself out of the rush and back to living from the "green zone" again.

Back to sleep. If you are churning out stress hormones and they are communicating to every cell in your body that you are not safe, your body does not want you to sleep deeply, as you need to be able to wake up quickly and save your own life. Your body has your best interests at heart. You just need to communicate to it that you are safe and that it is safe to sleep deeply and restoratively.

There is no more powerful way to activate the green zone, the PNS, than through your breathing. As stated previously, we activate the rest-and-digest arm of the nervous system through diaphragmatic breathing. Again, I know it might sound too simple to make a difference, but it truly does. You might have noticed that most adults today breathe from the top of their chest. If you watch, this is the only part of them that moves in and out. Adrenalin drives those short, sharp breaths. Diaphragmatic breathing communicates safety to your body. It is the fastest way to decrease both adrenalin and cortisol. Simply investing some time each day in focusing on how you breathe can truly be game-changing. I believe that not too long ago we lived from parasympathetic nervous system dominance, but now many people live in the "fight-

or-flight" response for the majority of the time, and we actually have to schedule time to live from that calming place. Schedule diaphragmatic breathing. I know from personal experience, and from observing others, that breathing truly is the cornerstone of calm which allows all of the "beauty bits" to be nourished.

You can switch over to the rest-and-digest arm of the nervous system through how you breathe, and also by decreasing, or omitting, caffeine and beginning to identify where you perceive pressure when you don't need to in your life. These shifts will help the SNS lose its dominant position in your nervous system, which for some of you will resolve your sleep challenges beautifully.

Other Factors

Any additional mechanisms that interfere with your body's ability to relax can lead to poor-quality sleep. Some of these additional factors include magnesium deficiency and worry.

Magnesium Deficiency

Magnesium and other minerals are critical for the body to physically relax, particularly the muscles. However, many people today don't consume enough magnesium. The body's magnesium requirements fluctuate, too, for when we are stressed and producing adrenalin, each unit of adrenalin that is made utilizes extra magnesium. This can lead to the muscles not having enough magnesium for sufficient relaxation.

For beautiful sleep, include optimal amounts of magnesium in your diet. Review the Beautiful Nutrients chapter for more information.

Worry

Another factor, discussed in the Stress Hormones chapter, which can play a role in someone not being able to sleep restoratively, is worry. You may be someone who worries about what others think. You may worry about things you have said or done over the day and what others said to you. You may worry about pleasing everyone in your life, and so you worry that you may have let someone down. What can you do about these things when you are lying in bed unable to sleep in the middle of the night? Nothing, unless you want to wake up the person on your mind. Accepting while you lie there in the dark that in that restless moment there is absolutely nothing you can do to clarify or rectify a situation that may or may not even exist can be a great start. My dear mum gave me a wonderful piece of advice about worrying. She suggested: "Don't worry about anything until it is a problem." That is such good advice. You can take it one step further if you like. Even if something is a problem, don't worry. Breathe. Face the situation or the person with your gorgeous, authentic self and be present in that moment. Life asks this of us at times.

As I mentioned in the Not-So-Beautiful Stress Hormones chapter, keeping the peace can also be a trait that leads to poor sleep. Review that information there if you feel you need to keep the peace. I want to help you see *why* you do it so that you can change your response, if it is hurting your health, especially if the stress hormone production triggered by your subconscious emotional responses won't allow you to deeply rest. And I want you to truly learn: there is no peace when you have to keep the peace.

By trying to keep the peace, you have no peace, and the impact on your nervous system tension, of always living in the red zone, can take a significant toll on your health. Realize that you don't have the peace you so desperately want by trying to keep the peace. With this new understanding you may find that you are able to gently and calmly have conversations with numerous people in your life that, before this insight, you would never have imagined yourself being able to do. Walking on eggshells doesn't serve you or the other person. Use your voice calmly and with good intention, as this may be your best sleep tonic.

RESOLVE SLEEP CHALLENGES

If you currently don't sleep restoratively, decide to make resolving this your focus for the next 30 days. Hopefully you are making notes in your journal as you progress through this book and are capturing what speaks to you. Take action in the area/s that resonated for you, as sleep is *critical* to every aspect of your inner health as well as your outer sparkle.

Kindness in words creates confidence.
Kindness in thinking creates profoundness. Kindness
in giving creates love.

Lao-Tzu

Chapter 8

Beautiful Posture and Movement:

the beauty of poise, grace, strength and flexibility

As Audrey Hepburn so elegantly said: "For beautiful eyes, look for the good in others; for beautiful lips, speak only words of kindness; and for poise, walk with the knowledge that you are never alone." Poise is, in itself, beautiful. It is way of carriage that communicates a deep appreciation for, and connection to, life and one's own self-worth. It is a way of holding yourself that doesn't get expressed when you feel unworthy or worthless on the inside. How you feel on the inside is reflected on the outside, and your posture is one way this is communicated.

POSTURE

This book doesn't seek to explore the history or the scientific literature relating to posture, nor does it go into detail about the biomechanics of your body; I simply want to acknowledge that many factors influence the posture you have today. Some of these factors include nutrition, the way you breathe, hydration, muscle mass, repetition of movement patterns, activity levels, as well as the emotional meanings you have attached to situations from the past.

Did you know, though, that the position of the spine in any moment can influence the emotions you feel in that same moment? Dr Donny Epstein, an incredibly gifted and passionate man who developed a treatment modality called network spinal analysis (NSA) and the author of numerous books, demonstrates powerfully through his work that the position of your spine can significantly influence your emotional responses to everything you experience in daily life. Have you noticed how, given an identical scenario, some people respond with an angry outburst while others respond with laughter? Sure, this response can be influenced by countless factors, but one you may not have considered is the position of your spine.

Try this. Hunch your shoulders over into a stooped position. Screw up your face so it feels tight. Clench your fists tightly closed. Tense your whole body. Now think of a situation that really makes you angry. It may be something you feel is unjust or a situation that unfolded 10 minutes or 10 years ago. Really think about whatever it is, while holding your body in the stooped, tense position described above. Let your body begin to vibrate with rage the more you focus on this thing that makes you angry. Focus intensely on what makes you angry while maintaining this posture. Now, in a split second, stand upright with your feet firmly connected to the ground, shoulder-width apart, and fling your arms wide open out to the side, open up across your chest, arch your back back a little, relax your face, smile widely, and open your eyes wide. Now focus on the thing that made you angry. Come on, focus on it! What you will notice is that you are unable to conjure the same level of anger towards what in the previous posture had you seething. You might not even be able to feel anger at all. Some of you might giggle when thinking about your anger situation with your spine in this new position.

I wanted you to experience that the way you hold yourself can influence everything from the way your body digests food and extracts and utilizes nutrients, to your skin, your mood, and the physical and emotional resources you bring to every situation you face in your life. Imagine that. Imagine being able to change how you respond to challenges through how you hold yourself and thereby shifting the messages your spine sends to your brain about what it perceives is going on for you.

Hold yourself structurally, knowing in your heart that you are worthy, worthy of life and of love, and decide to live with a graceful strength that inspires others to do the same.

MOVEMENT AND EXERCISE

When people think of exercise, they often link it to weight loss or weight maintenance, muscle-building or maintenance, strength, fitness level, flexibility, or "looking good". I want to encourage you to really consider the way you move and exercise, as movement is another avenue through which you can have a profoundly wonderful impact, not just on your body shape and size, but also on your physical and emotional health, your biochemistry, and your sparkle.

Choosing the Right Movement for You

Does exercise invigorate or exhaust you? Do you get the weight loss or weight gain results that you seek from your exercise? Does body fat seem to stay there no matter what you do? Do you build muscle easily? Reflecting on whether the way you move is actually doing what you want it to is worth some thought. Just as with nutrition information, we have been bombarded with what is the "right" way to exercise, and many people still mistakenly exercise with a commitment to the old adage "no pain no gain".

Yin and Yang Movement

As I have outlined in this book, as well as in *Accidentally Overweight* and *Rushing Woman's Syndrome*, many people now live constantly from the "red zone", always engaged in the fight-or-flight response. Given that humans have been on the planet for approximately 150,000 years, from an evolutionary perspective we have only been living in sympathetic nervous system (SNS) dominance for a relatively short period of time. (See, further, the Beautiful Sleep chapter.) In the past, the SNS only became dominant when we actually needed to save our own life. Once the threat to our life was over, we returned to living from the green zone (driven by the parasympathetic nervous system — PNS). Some people still have a balanced nervous system. If this is you, it means that you are readily able to switch between the SNS and the PNS appropriately. And for you, both what I call yang (intense) movement as well as yin (more breathing-focused) movement will serve you. However, if you are stuck in the rush of life, living on adrenalin and cortisol, relentlessly trying to juggle meeting everyone's needs and never your own, your nervous system will most likely be revved off the charts, constantly living from the red zone, even if you no longer notice that this is the case. If you then go and exercise with intensity, you run the risk of spending almost 24/7 in SNS dominance, depleting yourself further based on a mistaken belief about how you need to exercise to "get results". What if balancing your nervous system and incorporating more yin activity in your week supported your health goals, outcomes, and your shine? Here is how I learnt that this is possible.

Breathing as Messenger

I meet thousands of clients who, if the calorie equation were truly the only factor in weight loss, would be stick monsters (skinny), but they aren't. Countless women eat amazingly, even by my high standards, and move their bodies regularly with intensity; and they either stay the same size or, heaven forbid, their clothes just keep getting tighter. I met a lady a few years ago who trained for nine months for a marathon. She ran between 64 kilometres and 145 kilometres (40 miles and 90 miles) per week, every week for nine months. When she came to see me after she had completed the marathon, she showed me the diary she kept of her food consumption during this time, and it was clear she was burning far more fuel than she was consuming. Yet, over the nine months of training, she gained 12 kilograms (26 pounds).

I had my own experience with this, although the other way around. While I was doing my PhD, I was a runner. I would run daily, or at least six days a week. I would run for a minimum of one hour, but usually it was closer to two. I loved it. I was slim, happy, and healthy. And I ran that way because it was engrained in me that to maintain body shape and size, you had to burn far more than you ate.

However, when I became the programme manager in a beautiful health retreat, I had to leave home at 4.20am to get to work in time to cheerily wake the guests at 5.30am for their morning qigong practice (which is similar to t'ai chi). I left for work in the dark and arrived home in the dark, and I wasn't so obsessed with running that I was going to get up at 3am to go! So my exercise went from running one to two hours a day, to teaching 30 minutes of qigong — where you diaphragmatically breathe and gently move your arms — and taking the guests who hadn't exercised in a long time on what was called "the easy walk", 20 minutes on flat ground. I didn't break a sweat. My eating remained the same during this time. So, I went from burning bucket-loads of calories every day to burning far fewer calories ... and my clothes became looser and looser. This experience completely fried my brain, because I had been taught that precisely the opposite was supposed to happen.

It was this experience coupled with what I was observing in some, not all, of my clients that lead me to go back to my geeky biochemistry textbooks, determined to answer the questions: What leads the human body get the message that it needs to store fat, and what leads the human body to get the message that it needs to burn fat? And I wrote my first book, *Accidentally Overweight*, based on my findings.

It is not the training but your own body's response to that training that matters. In any given moment, your body is deciding which fuel to use, and it can only use two: glucose and/or fat. Humans can't use protein as fuel. We can break our proteins down into amino acids, which are then converted into glucose for the body to use. The decision on what to use is made based on the information the body is picking up from your environment about which fuel will best serve the preservation of your life in that split second. Glucose is your fast-burning fuel, the fuel for the SNS, the get-out-of-danger fuel that your body will use when it perceives your life is under threat, even if you are perfectly safe. Among other biochemical parameters, your body burns fat when the PNS is active, because it communicates to the body that you are "safe".

However, you can't use your thoughts to access the part of your nervous system that governs whether your SNS or your PNS is in charge. You can't instruct it the way you can "instruct" your arm to pick up a glass of water. The only way you can influence the message this part of the nervous system receives is via your breathing. When you breathe in a short, sharp, shallow way, this communicates to your nervous system that your life is in danger, as the only time you would have breathed this way historically was when it really was. But many adults breathe this way because of caffeine, the perception of pressure, or simply a lack of awareness. When we breathe diaphragmatically and slowly — pushing our lower abdomen ("belly") out with each inhalation and letting the tummy retract back in with each exhalation — your body perceives it is safe, because you wouldn't be able to breathe this way if your life were truly in danger.

What I worked out was that when I started doing and teaching qigong each day, I diaphragmatically breathed for 30 minutes daily, and my body's ability to burn body fat went to another level. When you live from the red zone, as so many people do these days, the body gets the message to predominantly burn glucose, not fat. When you have a balanced nervous system, you burn both fuels very efficiently.

My message to you is this: certain types of exercise can seem like more stress to an already over-stressed human body. Do you think our ancestors woke up and thought it would be a great day for a run? No. Back then, running meant we were attempting to escape from danger, while now it has become a way to burn off the excesses a Western lifestyle "affords" us. I'm not saying that running is bad, especially for those of you who love it and for those of you who feel energized, as opposed to exhausted, from it. Barefoot running, in particular, certainly promotes being present in the moment, and there is an incredible science that can be applied to running to promote fat-burning, not just so your clothes fit you. Burning body fat as opposed to constantly relying on glucose, also generates fewer free radicals and less inflammation, promotes nervous system calm, and great energy. I also know that for people who are what I call adrenally strong, usually because of the way they eat and their belief systems, they may find running brilliant, as it can help them burn off adrenalin created throughout the day. But when we are adrenally depleted from chronic stress, the hormonal profiles made by our endocrine system alter to one more likely to get the message that it needs to store fat.

While you may have believed that you were just exercising intensely, from your body's perspective, once the threat — perceived by your body to be present due to the release of stress hormones — is dealt with, the PNS slows our heart rate and respiration back down, brings the blood back to the digestive tract so that we can digest our food, works to repair any tissue damage, and increases libido. Isn't it clever? Night-time is when the parasympathetic nervous system is supposed to have plenty of time to do its job, provided we go to bed early enough. As you have read earlier, the sympathetic and parasympathetic systems are supposed to balance each other nicely, and in those people who have a balanced nervous system, high-intensity exercise will lead to fat loss, as the parasympathetic rest time between workouts is when muscle tissue is built.

Your Body's Feedback

Everyone is different. Please pay attention to what serves you. Let your body give you feedback, not your mind. Don't rely on what you have been told. Notice how you *feel* and respond with a type of movement that serves you. Be aware that needs change over time, too, depending on your base level of health and whatever else is going on in your life. If running and high-intensity exercise, combined with good eating, hasn't shifted your weight by now, it is not suddenly going to start doing so until some other work on your body's chemistry and nervous system is done.

Those who are unable to lose fat by doing regular high-intensity exercise may have a dominant sympathetic nervous system, and, consequently, an inhibited parasympathetic system. There is too much systemic stress coming from somewhere, and, for them, adding high-intensity exercise is counterproductive, as it adds to their sympathetic load, pushing them even more out of balance. Instead, you want to decrease the sympathetic load by reducing stressors and choosing an exercise that is done slowly and with the breath, such as restorative yoga, qigong, t'ai chi, yoga, or Feldenkrais. These activities will support the PNS and help balance the whole autonomic nervous system. The goal of so much of what I do to assist women's inner health, and therefore outer beauty, is to balance the nervous system so that when you do experience stress that is unavoidable, you cope very well; then you leave the stress, and all its health-depleting effects, behind.

In *Accidentally Overweight*, I discussed the importance of balance in your lifestyle and diet, but, as you can now see, the same also applies to exercise. If your life is stressful and you turn to a stressful form of exercise, such as intense cardio, you may encourage your body to burn glucose instead of fat stores. When your body is burning glucose you can tend to crave glucose and subsequently cravings for sugar, typically the refined type, increase. Who doesn't want the slow, even burn that occurs when you are accessing your fat stores? Just as there is an abundance of albeit well-meaning dietary information, you can also become overwhelmed when delving into the topic of exercise and how to move your body in a way that suits you. The answer truly lies with you. Please remember that it is your response to training, rather than the training itself, that is important.

Options

Incorporate exercise that you actually enjoy. If you don't like running, don't force it. Take a long stroll around the block, through a park, or by the sea instead. Appreciate your surroundings; enjoy the feeling of moving your body, noticing how the air feels on your face. Try a bike ride or an activity you have always wanted to try, such as a dance class. Even gentle movement will benefit your health, and if you enjoy it, you are more likely to continue on a regular basis.

Consider the expectations you place on yourself. So often I hear people say that they don't exercise because they used to be an athlete, or a runner, or at least a lot fitter than they are now. Their sheer frustration prevents them from doing any exercise. Start small if that feels good for you. Consider trying a form of exercise such as restorative yoga, Pilates, t'ai chi or any other activity that focuses on breathing. When you spend your day in SNS dominance, your body will be crying out for rest and repair (PNS activation). Remember, focusing on your breathing is the fastest, most effective way to activate your PNS, allowing your body to access its fat stores and stop craving sugar. The various forms of yoga can support your inner health and outer beauty physically, mentally, and spiritually, if you so choose, through the movement patterns but also through the breathing work. I am a huge fan. I am also deeply grateful for what a form of restorative yoga called Stillness Through Movement offers. The whole body is supported to truly rest; you change positions about every 20 minutes, and it is transformational for your health, especially your endocrine system, and hence your energy and sparkle.

Weight-bearing exercise is of particular importance, as it improves the strength of muscles and bones. Building muscle also increases your metabolic rate. Walking, hiking, dancing, skiing, and weight training are all examples of weight-bearing exercise. Exercising in the morning is an ideal way to wake up your body naturally. If this is not possible for you, or if you know you feel better exercising in the afternoon, then do that. Include at least one session of a relaxing style of exercise a week to help balance your nervous system. Start to make a conscious effort to move and breathe in a way that serves you and enhances your health.

Functional Movement

A concept I want to encourage you to explore is "functional movement". It is based on real-world situational biomechanics, which is not my area of expertise. I have, however, worked alongside pioneers in this field who possess the health, youthfulness, vitality, and physique that are testaments to these practices. The movement philosophy at the beautiful Gwinganna Lifestyle Retreat is based on functional and restorative movement. I simply want to introduce it to you, as I believe one of the focuses of movement needs to be on function. We are blessed to have bodies that give us the opportunity to enjoy and make the most of life, yet many people treat their body with no respect or gratitude for what it does for them and/or allows them to do.

We need to make sure that for our whole life, not just when we are young, our body is able to perform all the movements that are necessary for daily life and an active lifestyle. Imagine not being able to bend over and tie your own shoelaces in the second half of your life. Now imagine losing that independence, perhaps due to a lack of movement and/or poor dietary choices now. The way you eat, drink, think, move, perceive, and believe right now doesn't just impact on how you feel, function, and appear today. It will influence how you feel, function, and appear in the future as well.

Notice what movement patterns you need to run your life. For example, if you play tennis on the weekends, you want to make sure that your body is able to handle lunging, bending, jumping, and throwing. If you are parent, you need to be able to pick up your children, rotate with them, and then place them in their car seat, for example. Examine your lifestyle and activities and see what functions you need to be able to perform on a regular basis.

Seven Primal Movement Patterns

Every movement our bodies perform can be broken down into a series of one of seven movement patterns. These are often referred to as the Seven Primal Movement Patterns, and they are:

- squat
- lunge
- push
- pull
- bend
- twist
- gait

We all need a general functionality in each one of these patterns for normal daily life, such as loading groceries, lifting boxes, or running to catch the bus.

INNER NEEDS AND RHYTHMS

For your best shine, you want to be sure to build muscle from this point forward, or at minimum maintain your muscle mass where it is now. Don't lose muscle mass. It is a key driver of your metabolic rate, an efficient storage house for energy, and one way, along with dietary change, that we can help decrease our risk of developing type 2 diabetes. You want to learn about and practise functional movement, and also embrace restorative, breathing-focused practices, such t'ai chi and yoga. What image do you conjure up when you picture in your mind's eye a woman who has a long-term, regular yoga practice? In my experience, she typically looks more youthful than her chronological age, has long, lean muscles, and exudes a calm radiance, that is health-giving and beautiful. When you walk, or do any exercise, remain conscious of your inner needs and rhythms. The speed and distance you walk needs to serve your inner world, not a fantasy image of fitness. Expend the energy your body can happily give up, and this will change from day to day, year to year. And be sure to give your body as much rest as it needs to recover.

*Beauty announces the presence of love,
to which we are inherently drawn.*

Dr Libby

Chapter 9

Beautiful Skin, Hair and Nails:

a reflection of inner processes

Given that this is a book about beauty, I have decided to dedicate almost an entire chapter to beautiful skin, as the beauty question I am most frequently asked is: "How do I get beautiful skin?" Well, here is skin and skin care explained from all of the science, experience, observations, and intuition I have applied to date to help people have beautiful skin. What is nutritionally necessary to nourish hair and nails is also explained.

YOUR SKIN

Your skin is a barometer of what is going on inside your body, and all skin conditions, from psoriasis to acne to signs of aging, are the manifestations of your body's internal needs, including its nutritional ones.

The skin performs a multitude of tasks, most of which go unnoticed and under-appreciated. It protects us from disease and our daily exposure to particles in the air. It cools us when we are hot, and warms us when we are cold. It heals wounds inflicted on it, often without any assistance from us. It absorbs sunlight and produces vitamin D, which is critical to our bones and teeth, it keeps itself moist, slows its own aging, and every day attempts to renew and restore itself. While skin accomplishes all of this on its own, it still needs support in order to thrive, not just function. As Susan West Kurz so beautifully describes in her book, *Awakening Beauty*, with every blemish, rash, and wrinkle, the skin is asking us to understand its nature and support its efforts at self-renewal. Unfortunately, many of us respond to changes in our skin with practices that actually assault and injure it further, consequently accelerating the aging process, whether that is visible immediately or not. Still others do nothing for their skin, but nonetheless expect it to remain clear, beautiful, and youthful.

To help people change the way they consider and therefore treat their skin, I find it most powerful to help people understand what it does each day and how best to support its work. Skin is actually made up of three layers, which together are the perfect shield. The outermost layer, which is renewed each month, is the *epidermis* and this is the part you can see. The middle layer is the *dermis*, and below that is the foundation layer of the skin, known as the *subcutaneous layer*. All three layers work together to form healthy, vibrant skin.

Skin Structure and Growth

Epidermis

The epidermis itself is made up of layers, the top layer being the shield. As soft and supple as the skin can be, it is also a form of armour. Depending on your belief systems, you may perceive that it is a tough world out there and that you need protection from drying winds, rain, dust, as well as harsh words. The skin itself can handle all of that and a lot more.

The surface of the skin is made of dead skin cells that are flat and flexible. The cells that form the surface layer originate at the bottom of the dermis, a region known as the basal layer. Once they are born, these cells migrate upward to the surface. On their way, they are transformed into protein-producing cells called keratinocytes. Whenever the skin is cut or grazed, the keratinocytes signal the dermis to produce more cells so that the cut can be knitted together and the wound closed quickly. Isn't that amazing?

When they reach the surface of the skin and encounter air, the keratinocytes die and form a defence shield. After a week or two, they slough off, making way for another round of cells that form a new hard surface top layer. The journey from the basal layer to the surface of the skin takes about 28 days. This rate tends to slow to 35 days and even longer as we age.

Before they die, keratinocytes act with surrounding cells to produce chemicals that regulate your immune system. If you get scratched or cut, for example, these cells trigger an immune response to protect you from the bacteria that can enter through the open wound. Your immune system also helps cleanse the tissue of dirt and chemicals that infiltrate the opening. One of the consequences of an immune reaction is inflammation, characterized by the redness, swelling, and heat that surround a wound. Your immune system distinguishes your cells from foreign cells, assessing the foreign cells to determine whether they are dangerous to your health or not.

The more potentially harmful substances that enter your system, the more vigorously your immune system responds, and the more your tissues tend to inflame, resulting in more rapid aging. I believe that we need to do what we can to avoid using synthetic substances on our skin. The synthetic substances I choose to avoid include parabens, polyethylene glycols (PEGs), phthalates, and benzophenon. I also believe the skin loves it when we mimic its natural self and supply it with substances that nourish it. It is, after all, our largest organ.

I love the following phrase from Susan West Kurz: "Think of your epidermis as a living shield. It protects you from assaults from without while it guards the treasures within, among the most important of which is water." Well-hydrated skin maintains its plump, unlined youthfulness. Your epidermis makes sure your skin retains the moisture trapped within it, especially in the dermis. When the dermis is full of moisture, our skin is soft, dense, and pillowy. If it weren't for the epidermis, the moisture in your skin would come to the surface and evaporate, leaving your skin dry, wrinkled, and aged. By keeping the skin hydrated, the epidermis maintains your natural moisturizing factor, a term used in the beauty industry to describe skin moisture. According to Susan, the better your epidermis, the greater your natural moisturizing factor.

Skin varies in texture and sensitivity. It can be as tough as an old boot and as soft as a rose petal. One of the substances that give skin this beautiful quality is sebum, an oil-like compound that coats the epidermis. Sebum is made of fatty acids, fatty alcohols, waxes, lactic acid, and salts. These substances combine to give sebum a pH of between 4.3 and 6, which means it is slightly acidic. That is why the term "acid mantle" is used to describe the coating of the skin. This acid base on your skin is highly effective at neutralizing bacteria. Sebum also helps seal moisture into the skin.

The epidermis also contains the cells that provide pigment (colour) to the skin. These cells are called melanocytes and they make up only about two to three per cent of the cells in the epidermis. If the epidermis is treated with harsh chemicals and peels, the melanocytes can become deformed, and this can result in irregularities in skin colour.

From my research on skin health from a functional, anatomical, and biochemical perspective, here is my take on the physical processes vital to having a healthy epidermis. (The emotional aspects will be explored later.) Any programme that supports the epidermis also supports the health, youthfulness, and beauty of the skin. Substances that injure the epidermis, or strip it from the skin, are potentially playing a role in damaging or even destroying the skin, even though it may appear to give a short-term benefit. Alpha hydroxy acid, for example, strips the upper layers of the epidermis and exposes the soft tissue below. This may appear to enhance the skin's appearance for a short while, but it may actually accelerate the aging of the skin in the long term. There is a great divide in skin care approaches today. You either decide to work with the skin to assist it in doing what it does best, or you may end up injuring the skin, or replacing its normal function, for what I believe are short-term benefits.

Dermis

The dermis is a water world, and housed inside that wonderful world are blood and lymphatic vessels, small muscles, and nerves that convey our sense of touch. Wow! Doesn't that alone fill you with wonder? Also embedded in the dermis are sweat glands, hair follicles, and sebaceous glands, the glands that produce sebum. The body is constantly supplying the dermis with water to keep it moist, healthy, and beautiful.

Now here's some more incredible skin science. Traversing the dermis are fibrous strands, about 80 per cent of which are made of collagen, which is a protein. Collagen forms a dense matrix that protects the skin from splitting when it is pulled or twisted. The remainder of the strands are the elastin, another protein-based fibre. Elastin acts like rubber bands. Whenever the skin is pulled or stretched, elastin snaps it back into its original shape. As we age, the elastin tends to weaken.

Collagen and elastin are supposed to be moist and plump, which makes the skin appear full, soft, and unlined, typically how it appears in youth. Collagen and elastin give skin its fullness and shape. As we age, the fibres can be attacked by free radicals, which lead them to shrink and cross-link with other collagen strands, forming structures that, if you could see them, look like fish netting. As the collagen base shrinks, the skin at the surface folds over itself forming wrinkles. Sometimes the collagen becomes so cross-linked that the skin itself looks like fish netting. However, as you learnt in the Beautiful Foods and Beautiful Nutrients chapters, the antidote to the problem of free radicals is the antioxidants found in plants. So amp up the plant content of your diet.

Structurally, the dermis is infused with blood vessels that deliver oxygen and nutrients to nerves, glands, hair follicles, and cells, including those on the surface. When the body is cold, blood is supposed to start moving rapidly to bring in more warmth. When the body is hot, sweat glands start pumping moisture to the surface, where it evaporates and takes away some of the excess heat. Also within the dermis water world lie waste products that are constantly being expelled from your cells and tissues. These toxins are eliminated from your body by your lymph system. The lymphatic system is an extraordinary network of vessels and nodes that absorb intracellular waste from the gel-like lymph and take it away to be detoxified by the liver and expelled by the kidneys. Additionally, within the lymph vessels and nodes are antibodies and lymphocytes, which are cells of the immune system that gobble up foreign substances and therefore protect you from infection.

Just as with any waste removal system, the lymph works best when it is moving. When it is congested or blocked, waste can build up in the tissues, and this can cause blemishes, rashes, and irritations to the skin. Unlike your blood, which is pumped throughout the body by the heart, the lymph has no pump to help it keep moving. Its efficiency depends on you. You keep your lymph circulating through movement, such as walking, yoga, dance, and stretching. I am a huge fan of rebounding on a mini trampoline to stimulate the lymphatic system. It is a great way to improve energy: pop on a song, or three, that you love and bounce away. Often you can buy used rebounders on the internet. Or, if you'd prefer, do some calf raises. The better your lymph system is at removing waste, the clearer your skin will be.

One way to significantly reduce the burden on both your lymphatic system and your skin is to reduce, or omit, artificial substances from your diet. Many people don't do well focusing on eating less of anything, so instead focus on eating more … more real food, to really support health lymph and skin.

Deep within the dermis and down into the next layer, the subcutaneous layer, are hair follicles. The hairs that grow out of these follicles behave like reeds in a pond. In the same area as the follicles are the sebaceous glands, which produce sebum. Along with the skin's water content, sebum moisturizes the skin. Once secreted, the sebum attaches itself to hairs and climbs upward to the surface to create the skin's soft, yet protective, acid mantle. However, when the sebaceous glands are over-active, sebum can collect in the openings, or pores, of the skin, and in the places where the hairs appear at the surface. When this happens, pores and follicles may become blocked, infected and inflamed, causing blemishes, boils, swelling, and, potentially, scarring. Also buried within the dermis are the sweat glands that, as mentioned previously, release moisture to cool the body. Sweat glands also eliminate waste; they are one way we detoxify, and they function as an accessory to the work of the kidneys and urinary system.

Subcutaneous Layer

Directly below the dermis is the subcutaneous layer, which holds fats, muscle, and some blood vessels. The muscle and fat act as shock-absorbers for the skin, in a similar way to collagen. This is also the layer where we find bands of cellulite, which is essentially fat, and it is held in place by connective tissue lined with fat. Functions of metabolism also occur in this layer.

For me, Dr Rudolf Hauschka's philosophy about life, and particularly about the skin, deeply resonates. He taught that the beauty of your skin, and the cause of all skin challenges, could be revealed by understanding what he referred to as the threefold design of human beings.

We all have a nerve and sense function that enables us to think and provides us with sensory abilities. Each of us is blessed with organs that work through rhythmic action, or coordinated expansion and contraction, such as the heart and the lungs. Thirdly, we each have digestive and metabolic functions, including the ability to absorb nutrients for cellular activity — which is metabolism — and the capacity to eliminate waste. As Susan West Kurz so brilliantly describes: "the body is designed with the nervous system headquartered on the top floor, so to speak; the rhythmic system centred primarily in the chest where the heart and lungs are; and the digestive system in the middle and lower thorax, in the basement". These three systems permeate and integrate the activities of the body.

Here's what is even more special: that same threefold nature can be seen in the skin as well. As you now know, the upper layers are infused with nerve endings that tell us about the conditions in the environment. Our nerve and sense function has to lead the way if we are to be smart about what is going on around us. Just underneath our nerve function are our capillaries, which deliver oxygen and nutrients in the blood along with the cells of the skin and correspond to the heart and the lungs, the rhythmic organs. Below that are the lymph vessels and nodes, which as you have learnt carry waste away from the skin. As the waste disposal function, the lymph system corresponds to our digestion. So can you see why it spins my tyres that the threefold nature we find generally in the body also exists in the skin? Amazing.

In my experience, whenever skin breaks out in pimples, acne, or a rash, the origin of the problem will be found not in the skin itself, but in a waste disposal function of the body, typically the digestive system. When your body attempts to rid itself of excess waste that cannot be eliminated through the channels of preference for the body — mainly digestion, to which the liver is inextricably linked, and the kidneys — the skin steps in to assist in elimination. In other words, the skin believes it is helping you to be your healthiest self by getting rid of the waste. So rather than get frustrated at your skin for "betraying" you, understand that it is simply looking after you and, through that process, communicating to you that inner processes, such as digestion, liver, and/or the urinary system, need support. To have beautiful skin we must care for these systems, and please know that there is so much you can do to take even better care of them, as is outlined in the Beautiful Solutions chapter.

A Holistic View of the Face

With all of the structural and functional information about the skin having been shared, let me remind you that what tends to happen today when we consider the body, is that people see it in a fragmented way. People, and many health-care providers, often view body parts, or specific challenges, as separate from the whole. But I hope you can now appreciate that it is the overall health of your body, or, more accurately, your cells, that influences the appearance of your face and your skin. Clear, radiant skin is a reflection of great health, and, as you now understand, it is highly dependent on the optimal functioning of other systems, particularly digestion, the liver and the kidneys.

Again I reference the distinguished and highly valued work of Dr Hauschka and the numerous traditional medicine principles from numerous cultures that offer invaluable insight into the information the face offers us. For some, this exploration may not resonate; while, for others, it will offer what has potentially been a missing link in resolving skin challenges. It feels like common sense to me; in my work, I not only apply science to the functionality of the skin, but I also look to the location of congestion, to gain invaluable insight into the why for each person I work with. What follows is what I have observed.

For many, the places where blemishes and wrinkles appear on the face seem random. You may notice that you have a tendency to break out around your mouth or on your forehead, nose, or cheeks. In my experience, and once you truly understand how the skin works, you can see that these patterns are not random, but instead offer clues to a bigger picture. The face can be considered to be a precise map of the whole body, demonstrating where inner processes of specific organ systems may need support.

The Forehead

Remember the threefold explanation of the skin and the body as a whole? The forehead is believed to represent the senses and the nervous system, including thinking. If someone has an abundance of lines on the forehead, it may indicate that they spend too much time thinking and not enough time living from the heart, trusting their own instinct, and taking action. Blemishes and pimples on the forehead can also indicate excessive thinking that may be drawing vital energy away from digestive processes, taking away the robustness of a key elimination pathway, and allowing toxins to accumulate in the blood. Along with dietary change, part of my suggestion for this person will be to encourage them to find ways to stop worrying and thinking so much, and to relax more and enjoy life. Using the body more through sport or other physical activities can be highly beneficial for "forehead" people, assisting them in regaining their emotional balance. Coupled with digestive system support, remembering to trust your heart can be a pathway to beautiful skin.

The Middle Region, Including Under the Eyes

According to Dr Hauschka, and also in my experience, the area from the eyebrows to the bottom of this nose is a reflection of the "rhythmic system and related organs". Generally, the cheeks are considered to be a reflection of the lungs. Grey and sallow skin on the cheeks can indicate a degree of lung congestion and/or reduced oxygenation. Acne and other blemishes on the cheeks can reveal excesses of poor-quality fat and refined sugars that are adversely affecting the respiratory system. To help improve the oxygen content and circulation of the lungs, please pay attention to exposure to cigarette smoke, whether your own or that of others. Ideally, keep exposure to a minimum. Decrease, or eliminate, poor-quality fats such as trans fats, found in deep-fried foods, processed cakes and biscuits, and muesli bars. Many processed foods contain poor-quality fats. Amp up the green leafy vegetable content of your diet, especially the cruciferous vegetables described in the Beautiful Foods chapter. Many traditional medicine practices use these vegetables to specifically strengthen the health of the lungs. And walk daily, even if it is just for 20 minutes. Do more if you can. Increased respiration rates can help improve oxygen uptake and toxin expulsion, as the lungs are another way we eliminate substances our body doesn't want.

Below the eyes is an area that many women are challenged to keep looking firm and healthy. It is an area often referred to as the "eye bags", and it is associated with the health and function of the kidneys. This area of the face is home to the thinnest skin, and the skin sits closest to bone; as a result, it may react with swelling and fluid retention in a more visible way than any other part of the body would. Swelling may occur when the kidneys or urinary system need support and we are unable to effectively regulate the fluid content of our body. This can occur for a host of reasons, including a lack of restorative sleep. My observation is that the eye bags do not become swollen from drinking pure water. It is more likely to be due to other liquids, such as coffee, soft drinks (soda), processed juices (as opposed to fresh from a juicer), and/or alcohol. Do an experiment with yourself. Take a one-week break from coffee, alcohol, processed juice, and soft drinks, and notice the effect this alone has on your eye bags. Many people notice a significant change to their eye bags. The area below the eyes tends to become less lined and swollen, and the skin tightens and becomes more youthful. You can substitute weak black, or green, tea and still notice an improvement. On top of that, if you get more rest — at least seven hours a night if possible — your eye bags may shrink even further. If there are dark circles under the eyes, in my experience this is almost always resolved when digestion and/or liver health is addressed. For someone with significant dark circles under their eyes, there is often a food in this person's diet that doesn't serve them. Getting to the heart of this can completely resolve the dark circles, something I don't say lightly.

The bulb of the nose has long been associated with heart health. In many traditional healing modalities, the end of the nose is considered the gateway to the cardio-pulmonary system (your heart and lung systems). A swollen or red nose may indicate that the heart is somewhat overworked and needs support. I have seen this happen as a result of too much alcohol, too many poor-quality fats, quite often from processed foods and takeaways. Heartbreak or a perception of not being loved can also show up this way. The heart loves oxygen, and iron also assists with oxygen transport around the body. I have seen nose skin symptoms resolve when an existing iron deficiency is corrected. Minimizing consumption of the poor-quality fats in takeaway and processed food, as well as reducing intake of alcohol, refined sugar, and artificial ingredients can make a significant difference in this area. Taking a break from dairy products can often resolve nose skin symptoms. Further support heart health by amping up the plant content of your diet — the power of plants is endless. And you'd be surprised how making an effort to connect to the miracles around you and deeply appreciate your gift of life can impact your skin and your shine. Try it!

The Lower Region

I associate the region of the face from the nose to the chin as a reflection of the digestive system and the reproductive system. As I described in the Beautiful Digestion chapter, the digestive system can be thought of as a long tube beginning at the mouth and ending at the anus. In many traditional healing modalities, the bottom lip corresponds to the large intestine while the upper lip reflects the small intestine. If the lips are swollen, cracked, or particularly pale, these people do well consuming more warming foods and slow-cooked meals, high in plant content.

Just above the upper lip is the philtrum, the vertical indentation that can be a reflection of the health of the uterus. However, blemishes, swollen tissue, or lines in this area can indicate what traditional Chinese medicine refers to as "stagnation". It can be a sign that sex hormones are imbalanced — typically oestrogen dominance — and you may notice that the disturbances tend to disappear, or lessen, after menstruation. If they persist, it can indicate that the stagnation is chronic. The chin can also reflect the health of the reproductive organs. If the skin on the chin is dark or mottled, it can be a sign of long-term oestrogen dominance or the presence of fibroids, while blemishes on the chin or around the mouth can also indicate a sex hormone imbalance. To begin to resolve skin issues arising in this part of the face, focus on restoring sex hormone balance, as outlined in the Beautiful Solutions chapter.

Healthy Skin

The Power of Plants and Their Nutrients

The real food and nutrients that are of particular importance to all things beauty, such as vitamins C and E, are explained in the Beautiful Food and Beautiful Nutrients chapters; review those if you need to, so you know what roles these glorious foods and nutrients play. Please understand that no amount of topical nutrients can replace a lousy diet. But add some additional nutrients topically to a wonderful foundation of a real food way of eating, and you give the body and the skin everything they need for a flawless shine. Here is some skin-specific information to remind you, in bite-size pieces.

- The vitamins that are particularly good for the skin are vitamins A, C, E, K, and B complex. They all help improve the overall health of our skin, and they appear widely throughout real food.

- Among the most important new dermatological discoveries is the power of vitamins to help counter the effects of sun exposure. Research shows that appreciable photo-protection can be obtained from topical vitamins C and E. Additionally, research has demonstrated that supplementation with vitamin E at doses between 200 and 400 milligrams per day has been noted to reduce photo-damage and wrinkles, as well as improve skin texture.

- Further research showed a reduction of factors linked to DNA damage within skin cells when vitamins C and E were supplemented, leading researchers to conclude that antioxidant vitamins can help protect against DNA damage.

- Vitamins C and E help the skin by reducing the damage caused by free radicals, which are generated by many things, including increased respiration, and exposure to smoke and pollution. Free radicals gobble up collagen and elastin, the fibres that support skin structure, leading to wrinkles and other signs of aging. Good food sources of vitamin C include citrus fruit, capsicum, and kiwifruit, while vitamin E is found in nuts, seeds, and eggs yolks.

- When dietary levels of vitamin A drop too low, you are likely to see some skin-related symptoms, including a dry, flaky complexion and/or scalp. That is because vitamin A is necessary for the maintenance and repair of skin tissue. Orange vegetables are rich in beta-carotene, which your body converts to vitamin A.

- When it comes to skin, one of the most important nutrients is biotin, one of the B-group vitamins. Biotin forms the basis of skin, nail, and hair cells. Without adequate amounts, you may have dermatitis, an itchy, scaly skin reaction, or sometimes even hair loss. Even a mild deficiency can cause symptoms. Most people get enough biotin without even trying if they eat a real food diet, as it is widely spread throughout real food. However, if people rely too much on processed foods for too long, deficiency can result. Food sources include bananas, eggs, and brown rice.

- Niacin, another B vitamin, can help the skin retain moisture, and it also has anti-inflammatory properties to soothe dry, irritated skin.

- Zinc is a mineral your skin loves and needs. It is particularly important if you have acne. Acne itself can be a symptom of a zinc deficiency. Eaten in food or taken as a supplement, zinc works to help clear skin by taming oil production and may be effective in controlling the formation of acne lesions or help those already on your skin to clear sooner. Food sources of zinc include oysters (preferably grown in water uncontaminated with heavy metals), red meat (preferably organic), and seeds, particularly sunflower seeds and pumpkin seeds.

- Alpha-lipoic acid acts as a powerful antioxidant and supports vitamins C and E, as well as doing its own wonderful work. I love what I have seen it do to skin.

- Essential fatty acids (EFAs) are the rock stars of the skin world. Fats from whole foods help to beautifully nourish your skin. If your skin is dry, prone to inflammation, and frequently dotted with white heads and black heads, you may be lacking EFAs, nutrients that are crucial to the production of the skin's natural oil barrier. Without an adequate supply of EFAs, the skin produces a more irritating form of sebum, or oil, which can result in congestion. Cracked heels are another sign of EFA deficiency. Balancing your intake of omega-3 and omega-6 fats is part of the solution. Most people consume too many pro-inflammatory omega-6 fats from processed foods. The type of omega-6 fat in evening primrose oil, however, is very good for hormone balance and skin. The omega-3 fats are often lacking. They are found mostly in: cold-water oily fish, including salmon and sardines; flaxseed; hemp and chia seeds and their oils; as well as in walnuts. Omega-3 oils go rancid easily, so they must be kept in the fridge and consumed alongside an antioxidant-rich diet (high in plants). I love food-based oil supplements that combine these oils, and I have seen them significantly improve skin softness and texture. Coconut and its oil, consumed and applied topically, can also be highly beneficial to skin.

Tips for Beautiful Skin

You can support the skin in other simple ways, listed below.

- Don't smoke. Avoid tanning beds and excessive sun bathing. All three age your skin prematurely.

- Don't rub your eyes; use a light touch on your face always. If your eyes get itchy, apply a cold compress.

- Keep your hands off your face! Because your hands touch so many surfaces, they carry dirt and germs. Rub your eyes, stroke your chin, cup your cheek, and you have transferred everything on your hands to your face. As an extension of this, use headphones or a headset when talking on the phone. This, too, helps keep hands and germs away from your face.

Skin Problems

Acne

The processes involved in acne can be common to other skin challenges. From my perspective, healing acne is different from treating acne; it is important to first understand the precise process that creates acne, for then you can see why I suggest what I do to heal it. Acne arises when the sebaceous glands become over-active and sebum collects and blocks hair follicles and pores. As the keratinocytes migrate upward from the lower levels of the skin, they get bogged in the sebum. These cells don't live for very long, so soon they die, and they become trapped in the follicles and pores. The excess sebum and dead cells form a plug, or a blackhead, in the pore, which prevents the usual drainage of the oil. As the excess sebum accumulates, bacteria collect in large populations and feed on the sebum. They also irritate the skin and eventually cause infections, which combine to form a pustule or a pimple. Other factors are involved as well. Sex hormone imbalances increase the production of sebum, which tends to mean more blocked pores and infections, which in turn create pustules and rashes of acne.

Almost always, poor digestive function is the first trigger. Poor digestion adds a load to the liver and kidneys; they aren't able to filter the higher levels of hormones in the blood efficiently, and the hormones stimulate additional sebum production. I have seen countless cases of acne improve and then resolve with a commitment to caring for and supporting the digestive system, liver, and kidneys, suggestions for which are presented in the Beautiful Solutions chapter. Emotionally, acne can be challenging. Most people with acne will say to me that they dislike themselves. They have expanded the dislike that would have initially been for the pustules to themselves as individuals, and I work to help them see that what they feel is a wound or an immense frustration for them (their skin) can become a gift, for it is almost always our body trying to wake us up to eat, drink, move, think, believe, or perceive differently. And sometimes those beliefs are about ourselves, about who we are. Some precious people have forgotten that they are precious and they can no longer see their own beauty. I find if the person can accept where they are (and I know that is a big ask) and begin to work with what is — and if we can get them eating in a way that serves them as an individual, along with some liver support — improvements in the skin begin. And this is so encouraging for the person.

Additional Factors in Aging

In addition to oxidative stress, telomere shortening and increased glycation have also been linked to aging. What does this mean and what can we do about it?

Oxidative stress: To remind you, a major cause of aging is oxidative stress. It is the damage to DNA, proteins, and lipids (fatty substances) caused by oxidants, which are highly reactive substances containing oxygen. These oxidants are produced normally when we breathe, and also result from inflammation, infection, and the consumption of alcohol, cigarettes, and other pollutants. We have explored, in depth, the power and importance of antioxidants — found in your coloured plant foods — to neutralize the effects of oxidative stress.

Telomeres: Inside the centre or nucleus of a cell, our genes are located on twisted, double-stranded molecules of DNA called chromosomes. At the ends of the chromosomes are stretches of DNA called telomeres, which protect our genetic data, making it possible for cells to divide. Telomeres have been compared with the plastic tips on shoelaces because they prevent chromosome ends from fraying and sticking to each other, which would scramble our genetic information and possibly lead to disease or death. Telomeres are in place to prevent this. Yet, each time a cell divides, the telomeres get shorter. When they get too short, the cell can no longer divide and it becomes inactive or dies. This is one of the processes associated with aging. An enzyme named telomerase adds bases to the ends of telomeres to counteract their shortening. In young cells, telomerase keeps telomeres from wearing down too much. But as cells divide repeatedly, there is not enough telomerase, so the telomeres grow shorter and the cells age. Telomerase remains active in sperm and eggs, which are passed from one generation to the next. If reproductive cells did not have telomerase to maintain the length of their telomeres, we would potentially become extinct.

While telomere shortening has been linked to the aging process, it is not yet known whether shorter telomeres are just a sign of aging (like grey hair) or actually contribute to aging. What scientists are starting to understand is that antioxidants potentially play a role in slowing telomere shortening — yet another reason to amp up the real food, particularly plant, content of how you eat.

Glycation: Another factor in aging is glycation. This occurs when glucose (sugar) from what we eat binds to some of our DNA, proteins, and lipids, leaving them unable to do their jobs. If we have a diet high in processed foods, the problem becomes worse as we get older, since the cumulative sugar intake for most just keeps growing. This can cause cells and tissues to malfunction, resulting in aging, or in some cases disease. Not that long ago in human evolution, processed, high-sugar foods didn't exist. Then, in the not-too-distant past, they were eaten only on special occasions, like birthday parties, but now they have become part of every day for too many people. I cannot say this enough: it is what you do every day that impacts on your health, not what you do sometimes. The aging process will potentially be slowed if you consume less refined sugar.

The Emotional Approach to Skin

I am driven to help people literally get to the heart of their health matters. As you now understand, I believe that the so-called markers of beauty — such as your skin, hair, and nails — are simply a barometer for inner processes doing their best to wake you up to eat, drink, move, think, believe, or perceive in a different way than you are doing now. When you can see an outer beauty challenge as a gift from your body, even though that is the last thing it feels like when you are in the midst of an acute or chronic beauty challenge, it can open you up to explore your health and beauty in a new way.

For many people today there is a fear and anxiety within them, often centred on whether they are (good) enough, which we will explore in the Beautiful Insights chapter. The emotion of anxiety can only be present if you are focused on the future. I find depressed emotions can only be present if you focus on the past. If you are present, there is only peace. That may sound like a cliché, but think about it. It is an accurate description.

Louise Hay teaches that thoughts and beliefs you may or may not be aware of can lead to dysfunctions in your physical health. Sometimes I ask a client whether they feel a particular emotional state or phrase resonates for them, based on Louise's work or my own intuition. I sometimes find that the client does feel a certain way or that the phrase does speak to her, and this leads us to an insight that can often have a wonderful impact in many areas of her life.

I share a few skin conditions here to show you how they might be emotionally explored. Please understand that there are almost always physical processes such as dietary change that need to occur for these skin conditions to heal. And for many people, dietary change is all they need. However, for some people dietary change generates significant improvements but not resolution. So I am offering you this additional information as some people need the emotional insight for the skin challenge to resolve. If any of the concepts below resonate for you, enquire within, perhaps using a journal, and explore whether these perceptions still serve you, or whether they are based on a story you made up a long time ago about who you are.

Skin Problems

When it comes to what Louise refers to as "skin problems", she suggests that you explore if you are anxious or fearful. She describes skin issues as being related to "old, buried guck", or a perception that you are threatened.

Rashes

For rashes, Louise suggests you explore "irritation over delays", and asserts that for an adult it is "a babyish way to get attention".

Psoriasis

For psoriasis, try on a "fear of being hurt. Deadening the senses of the self. Refusing to accept responsibility for our own feelings." There are dietary suggestions and other support ideas for psoriasis in the Beautiful Solutions chapter.

Vitiligo

According to Louise, the feeling behind vitiligo is "feeling completely outside of things. Not belonging. Not one of the group." Please remember that this is the person's *perception*, not necessarily how you may see the life of someone with vitiligo. This perception needs exploring as, in my experience, it has always been a story someone made up so that they could feel "safe". I have seen that this emotional exploration, coupled with a diet excluding either casein (one of the proteins in dairy food) and/or gluten (found in wheat, rye, oats, barley and triticale), also makes a difference.

Eczema

In almost every case of significant, chronic, unresolved eczema, there is a rage at a masculine presence in that person's life, quite often the father. I could share literally hundreds of stories with you. The relationship with this man may now be enjoyable or comfortable or just improved from where it was, but there is still a rage — not just an anger — toward him. And sometimes, horrific traumas have occurred to lead to that. But trauma and sadness can be resolved.

Compassion here is vital — Nelson Mandela is testament to that. Some of the most moving stories I have ever heard involve someone turning a horrific hardship into their greatest gift or opportunity. As Donny Epstein wisely says: "The greater the wound, the bigger the gift." If you have significant, chronic, unresolved eczema, explore with curiosity, rather than anger or fear, whether any of this resonates for you. If it doesn't, cast this aside. If it does, let yourself scream at the wall and then cry the tears you are aching to shed, see the situation(s) that hurt you with adult eyes, rather than continuing to consider this person through the lenses of your younger self, when your rage began. Couple this with the dietary and fatty acid suggestions in the Beautiful Solutions chapter, and take care of yourself. Love yourself the way you perceive he never did.

Human hair is made of keratin, which is made from amino acids, and dead skin cells. Its primary function is to prevent heat loss from a person's head. It also acts as an excretory mechanism for the body.

While I was doing my PhD examining nutritional and biochemical factors in children with autism spectrum disorder (ASD), a study was published by another research group which had assessed the heavy metal content of hair from children who went on to develop ASD, compared to those who didn't develop any conditions before the age of five. The initial conclusion from the study was that heavy metals were not involved in the aetiology of ASD, as the children with ASD had significantly lower levels of heavy metals in their hair, compared to the control group. However, a number of years later, after additional research, the scientists retracted their original conclusions and released a new statement about what their research meant. They said that children without ASD had higher levels of heavy metals in their hair as they were able to excrete them from the body more efficiently than children with ASD, and that children with ASD potentially had higher levels of heavy metals stored in their body, unable to use the hair as a mechanism of excretion as affectively as children without ASD. This research was a great reminder to me that the body works to excrete the substances it doesn't require or those that may be toxic at high levels. Hair is one way our body does this.

Hair Structure and Growth

The composition of the hair is made up of two separate structures: the follicle in the skin and the shaft we see. The follicle is a stocking-like structure that contains several layers with different roles. A projection forms at the base of each follicle and, if you could see it, it looks like a finger being pushed a small distance through the bottom of a stocking. This projection is called a papilla and it contains tiny blood vessels that feed the cells. The living part of the hair is the bottom part of the stocking surrounding the papilla. This is called the bulb. The bulb is the only part fed by the capillaries. The cells in the bulb divide every 24 to 72 hours, faster than any other cells in the body.

The follicle is surrounded by an inner and outer sheath. These sheaths protect and shape the growing hair shaft. The inner sheath follows the hair shaft and ends below the opening of a sebaceous gland and sometimes an apocrine (scent) gland. The outer sheath continues all the way up to the gland. A muscle attaches below the gland to a fibrous layer around the outer sheath. When this muscle contracts, it causes the hair to stand up.

The sebaceous gland is important because it produces sebum, which, just as it is for the skin, behaves like a natural conditioner for the hair. More sebum is produced after puberty, while many women will describe a turning point at varying ages or after very challenging times, when they notice sebum production starts to decrease.

The hair shaft is made up of dead, hard protein called keratin in three layers. The inner layer is called the *medulla* and it isn't always present. The next layer is the *cortex*, and the outer layer is known as the *cuticle*. The cortex makes up the majority of the hair shaft. The cuticle is formed by tightly packed "scales" in an overlapping structure similar to roof shingles. Most hair-conditioning products attempt to affect the cuticle. Pigment cells are distributed throughout the cortex and medulla giving the hair its colour.

Hair on the scalp grows about 0.3 to 0.4 millimetres per day or about 15 centimetres (six inches) per year. Unlike other mammals, for humans hair growth and loss is random and not seasonal or cyclic. At any given time, a random number of hairs will be in various stages of growth and shedding, and there are three stages of hair growth known as catagen, telogen, and anagen.

The *catagen phase* is a transitional stage, and three per cent of all hairs are in this phase at any time. The duration of this phase is about two to three weeks. During this time growth stops and the outer root sheath shrinks and attaches to the root of the hair. This is the formation of what is known as a club hair.

The *telogen phase* is the resting phase and accounts for 10 to 15 per cent of all hairs. This phase lasts for about 100 days for hairs on the scalp, and much longer for hairs that make up the eyebrows, eyelashes, arms and legs. During this phase the hair follicle is completely at rest and the club hair has completely formed. If you pull out a hair in this phase, it will reveal a solid, dry, white material at the root. About 25 to 100 telogen hairs are typically shed each day.

Anagen is the described as the active phase of the hair. The cells in the root of the hair divide rapidly at this stage. A new hair forms and pushes the club hair up the follicle and eventually out. During this phase the hair grows about 1 centimetre every 28 days. Scalp hair stays in this active phase of growth for two to six years. If people have difficulty growing their hair beyond a certain length, it can be due to a short active phase of growth, while people whose hair seems to grow quickly and easily, tend to have a longer active phase of growth. The hair on the arms, legs, eyelashes, and eyebrows have a very short active growth phase of about 30 to 45 days, which is the reason why they are so much shorter than scalp hair.

Straight Hair and Curly Hair

The cross-sectional shape of hair determines the amount of natural curl it has. The more circular the shaft is, the straighter the hair is, while the more elliptical the shaft, the curlier or kinkier the hair. The cross-sectional shape also determines the amount of shine the hair has. Straighter hair tends to be shinier because sebum can travel down the hair more easily. The curlier the hair, the harder it is for the sebum to travel down the hair, which can lead to dryness.

Healthy Hair

Like all of the other aspects of beauty, healthy hair is firstly dependent on great digestion, particularly protein digestion. If this is a challenge for you, review the Beautiful Digestion chapter as well as the digestion support strategies in the Beautiful Solutions chapter. I have also found that when undesirable changes to the hair are occurring, the adrenals usually need support, outlined in detail in the Beautiful Solutions chapter.

Nutrition

All nutrients contribute in some way to the health of the hair. Some specific examples include:

- Split ends are the result of the dead cells that make up the hair flaking apart; vitamin C and EFAs have been shown to slow down the formation of split ends and help hair that breaks easily.

- If hair becomes finer over time, this tends to be the result of the hair follicle shrinking. Vitamin D plays a critical role in the healthy function of the hair follicle.

- If the hair seems to become becomes oily out of the blue, sex hormone balance usually needs to be addressed.

- If the hair becomes dry out of the blue, more essential fatty acids are usually needed in the diet. If this does not rectify the dryness in about six weeks, it may be worthwhile investigating thyroid function.

YOUR NAILS

Fingernails and toenails are important structures made of keratin, which have two distinct purposes. Nails act as protective plates and enhance sensations of the fingertip. The fingertip has many nerve endings in it, allowing us to receive volumes of information about objects we touch. The nail acts as a counterforce to the fingertip, providing even more sensory input when an object is touched.

Nail Structure and Growth

The structure we know of as the nail is divided into six specific parts: the root, nail bed, nail plate, eponychium (cuticle), perionychium, and hyponychium. Each of these structures has a specific function, and if disrupted can result in an abnormal-appearing fingernail. Nutrients also play a role in the appearance of nails.

The root of the fingernail is known as the germinal matrix. This portion of the nail is actually beneath the skin behind the fingernail and extends several millimeters into the finger. The fingernail *root* produces most of the volume of the nail and the nail bed. This portion of the nail does not have any melanocytes, the melanin- (colour-) producing cells. The edge of the germinal matrix is seen as a white, crescent-shaped structure called the lunula, which can become smaller or disappear due to poor digestion and/or low mineral intake.

The *nail bed* is part of the nail matrix. It extends from the edge of the germinal matrix, or lunula, to the hyponychium. The nail bed contains blood vessels, nerves, and melanocytes. As the nail is produced by the root, it streams down along the nail bed, which adds material to the undersurface of the nail, making it thicker. Minerals such as calcium, magnesium and boron contribute to this. It is important for normal nail growth that the nail bed be smooth. If it is not, the nail can split or develop visible grooves.

The nail plate is the actual fingernail, made of translucent keratin. The pink appearance of the nail comes from the blood vessels underneath the nail, and these will become pale when there is iron deficiency. The underneath surface of the nail plate has subtle grooves along the length of the nail that help anchor it to the nail bed. The *eponychium* or *cuticle* is situated between the skin of the finger and the nail plate fusing these structures together and providing a waterproof barrier, for which the essential fatty acids are crucial.

The *perioncyhium* is the skin that overlies the nail plate on its sides. It is also known as the paronychial edge. The perionychium is the site of hangnails and ingrown nails, while the *hyponychium* is the area between the nail plate and the fingertip. It is the junction between the free edge of the nail and the skin of the fingertip, also providing a waterproof barrier.

Nails grow all the time, but their rate of growth slows down with poor circulation, digestion and nutrition. Fingernails grow faster than toenails at a rate of approximately 3 millimetres per month. It takes six months for a nail to grow from the root to the free edge. Toenails grow about 1 millimetre per month and take 12 to 18 months to be completely replaced.

Healthy Nails

Nutrition

Nails are mostly made up of amino acids, which are the building blocks of protein. They also have minerals built in to their matrix, including calcium, magnesium, boron and zinc. Including adequate protein in your diet is essential to nail quality, and often very soft nails are the result of poor protein utilization in the body, which can be due to poor intake or poor digestion. Changes in fingernail appearance can indicate that something deeper is going on in the body. They can provide clues to your health and nutritional status. If your nails aren't what you want them to be, use it as a signal from your body that the way you eat, drink, move, think, believe, or perceive needs to change. Nails can, after all, be a reflection of bone health so resolving a nail challenge now may assist bone health in the future.

The key to creating truly strong, healthy nails is nourishment. Just because you eat a specific food or nutrient doesn't mean you get it. Much of sparkling health comes down to the way you absorb and utilize nutrients in the body. Therefore, the first step in great quality nails is outstanding digestion. If this is a challenge for you, review the Beautiful Digestion chapter as well as the digestion support strategies in the Beautiful Solutions chapter.

Secondly, as you now understand, nail growth is considered to be a "non-vital" process; they are not necessary to save your life if it was being threatened. So stress not only takes away from key digestive processes, which can impact on nail health, but also the nutrients the nails need are more likely to be used in the creation of stress hormones and other aspects of the get-out-of-danger response than they are to be sent to nourish the nails. Therefore, restorative practices such as t'ai chi and restorative yoga — anything that promotes diaphragmatic breathing — fosters the mechanisms that allows your beauty bits, including your nails, to be supported. Understand the stress mechanisms more from the blog posts available at: www.drlibby.com/bioresources

Tips for Improving Nail Health

A range of nail challenges is specifically addressed in the Beautiful Solutions chapter. Here are some general tips for great nail health.

- Peeling cuticles may be an indication of iron or essential fatty acid deficiency. Address this while also rubbing a little coconut oil around your nail beds each evening.

- Explore you biochemistry and get some thorough blood tests, as nail health can be affected by iron deficiency, B_{12} deficiency or essential fatty acid deficiency.

- Increase your consumption of zinc-rich foods, as white spots on your nail can be a sign you may be zinc-deficient. Good sources include nuts, seeds, and red meat.

- Love for your liver! Who would have thought your liver function can be reflected in your nail health? Pale, brittle or weak nails can be an indication that your liver needs some love. Incorporate more of the brassica group of vegetables, such as broccoli, kale and cauliflower.

- Give your body and nervous system a chance to repair. If your body perceives that it is constantly in danger, the last thing it will want to maintain is healthy nails. Do at least one thing every day that is restorative for you, such as yoga, diaphragmatic breathing or simply lying with your legs up the wall for five minutes.

An Additional Consideration

These days it is possible to obtain "fake" versions of beauty bits that we may not be satisfied with. If we are dissatisfied with our nails, for example, it is common for people to have their nails covered over. There is absolutely nothing wrong with this — it can be fun and bring you great pleasure, so by all means do it. But I cannot encourage you enough to also work on your nail health from the inside out. Your nails can be a reflection of numerous interior processes, including protein metabolism and bone health. If these issues aren't addressed, my concern is that more significant health challenges could become apparent in the future. So by all means enjoy your beauty salon nails, but focus on supporting your own nail health at the same time. Challenges with beauty bits can light the way to better health.

Understanding that your skin, hair and nails are an exterior demonstration of what is going on inside you, helps you to know where to begin if you'd like to make changes or if your body is asking you to makes changes by giving you certain signs. Treat yourself with the love and compassion you deserve and see challenges in these areas not as stumbling blocks that interfere with your joy in life, but rather as the guiding light that they are.

Our deepest fear is not that we are inadequate. Our deepest fear is that we are powerful beyond measure. It is our light, not our darkness that most frightens us. We ask ourselves, 'Who am I to be brilliant, gorgeous, talented, fabulous?' Actually, who are you not to be?

Marianne Williamson

Chapter 10

Beautiful Insights:

a love letter for you

Would you believe me if I told you that your experience of your own beauty is entirely dependent on you loving you? I don't mean in a conceited way. Nor do I mean that you just need to affirm that you love yourself and it's a done deal. Every human's greatest fear is that they are not (good) enough, and as a result that they won't be loved. We are born this way. It is Human Psychology 101. Without love a human baby dies, as someone has to care for us enough to feed us. Other animals can forage for food and find shelter and survive. So this is not some artificial construct that develops over time — it is hardwired into our nervous system at our most fundamental level. A condition called "failure to thrive" has sadly been observed in babies who don't receive food and love. So we are born with the belief that love is essential to our survival. And in the early years it is. We can't find our own food, clothing, and shelter, the basics of human survival. Yet as adults, while a life with love in it is delicious, love is not actually physically *essential* for survival. We can now obtain food, clothing, and shelter for ourselves. However, many adults still live as though love is still essential to their survival, and this has an impact on every decision they make, and therefore their choices and behaviour. Let me show you how.

BELIEFS AND BEHAVIOURS

Creating Our Own Meanings

My favourite author, Geneen Roth, says, "We all follow life instructions given to us 10 or 30 or 50 years ago by people we wouldn't ask for street directions from today." We have created meanings from what was going on around us at a very young age, only we didn't know that this is what we were doing. We simply thought that when Dad had "that" look on his face, it meant he was happy or sad or angry or about to explode. And when Mum made "that" sighing sound, it meant that she was disappointed or tired, relieved or in her happy place. We created those meanings. In these situations, our mother and father hadn't told us with words that they felt a certain way. Nor did we approach them and enquire: "You know that sigh sound you just made, Mum? Did you mean

I'd disappointed you by not putting my dirty dishes in the sink? Or did it mean that you feel relieved that dinner is over in our rowdy household and very soon you'll be relaxing in front of the TV, so it was more of a relieved sigh? Could you please clarify the meaning of your sigh for me, Mum?" We don't do that. We simply observed these people whose love and attention we want more than anything else in the whole world at that age, as well as the environment, and we formed beliefs about how the world is and who we must be within that world. Yet this is *our* version of the world, which is why, when you speak to twins about their lives growing up, you can wonder whether they have come from the same family.

I have listed some examples below to help you make sense of this concept. "Don't be so full of yourself — people don't like that" can eventually, if we hear it enough times, become the belief that "If I want to be loved and accepted, I need to be dull and dim, and dumb myself down." Another example. If we see our parents arguing about money, if money is a source of conflict in our families, or if no one ever talks about it, we give meaning to those situations in the form of beliefs: "If I want to be happy in a relationship, I'd better not talk about, nor think about, nor ever bring up the subject of money."

Translating Beliefs to Behaviours

As humans, we come to understand situations by giving them meaning. And out of these meanings, beliefs are created, which once formed, become the template for how we see ourselves and also how we behave, because your behaviour is the outermost expression of your beliefs. We then spend the rest of our lives acting as though our subjective beliefs — beliefs you have created, but you don't realize you have — are reality itself. ("I will never have enough", "I must keep the peace", "I am lazy/dumb/unlovable, if I am not 'slim', if I am not 'beautiful'," "If I don't please people and say yes whenever anyone asks me to help them, then I won't be loved.") We believe that the way we see our situation is the way things are, and that there is no other way. And our actions follow accordingly.

Most of us don't even know what we believe. We are convinced of the rightness of what we see and feel, that we don't realize that we see things as *we* are, not as *they* are. It never occurs to us that our belief system is subjective, and that there are dozens of ways to interpret the same situation. I cannot encourage you enough to begin to name and recognize the extent to which your own version of reality is based on comments made and instructions given to you "by people you may not even ask for street directions today". If you don't enquire within yourself about this, then your perception of who you are, how you appear, your emotional, financial and spiritual life remains frozen in the past, hijacked by beliefs that, for the most part, are out of alignment with, and have no relevance to, your current ideals and values and the adult you have become.

Updating Beliefs and Behaviours

Affirmations — and Limitations

As much as I love positivity and optimism — and I consider myself to have both of these traits — I have not found that it is possible to completely replace one set of beliefs with another by only using what have become known as "affirmations". Of course they can help. They help shift your focus to one of positivity, and they help you have hope that life can be better and that situations can change. But you can repeat "I am lovable" a thousand times a day, you can put "I am beautiful" in your car, on your mirror, your computer screen, inside your glasses if you like, but if an earlier belief or conviction of being unlovable or not beautiful is installed in your psyche based on beliefs you created before you could talk, you will only feel better for a moment, because you won't actually believe it yourself.

If you don't do the actual work of deconstructing your fundamental beliefs, the affirmations have no place to land or stick, and their impact is unlikely to be lasting. By all means do affirmations — they can be nourishment for your soul. It's just that I have yet to meet someone for whom they alone dismantled what was laid down at the beginning of their time on Earth. Of course be positive and affirm that you are loved and appreciated and beautiful. Just explore your beliefs as well for lasting, sustained change, and so that you truly, madly, deeply fall more and more in love with yourself with every breath you take.

The Action–Belief Interaction

When people say things like "Your beliefs determine your experience", think about this: if you believe that there aren't enough hours in the day or if you believe in being poor or that you will always be fat, that will be your experience. In other words, when you look through "shattered" lenses, the world looks "shattered". It has always been true that you act according to your beliefs, and, since the way you act has consequences, your beliefs manifest in the world through a variety of situations. When you act out your beliefs, you see the results of your actions everywhere. It is precisely what happens when you buy a certain coloured car of a specific make and model, you suddenly see those cars everywhere, don't you? Well, guess what? They have always been there; it is simply that now a part of your brain, called the reticular activating system, is primed to notice them. Beliefs work the same way. You see "evidence" of what you believe everywhere, and you never notice the zillions of examples that make those beliefs null and void.

Reclaiming Beauty

Clearly it is taking different actions, not just naming beliefs, that leads to change, but in my experience with human health, self-love, and radiant beauty, achieving long-lasting change is impossible without first becoming aware of the deep-seated convictions that are driving your behaviour. If you don't realize that the way you are seeing things is not the way they are, if you don't understand that you see yourself, how you appear to others, your family, your relationships with food, money, and the world through a version of reality that you developed before you could talk, you believe there is no other way to see and consider the world. You only know what you have experienced, and therefore those around you must be delusional if they describe it or you any other way.

You were born knowing you are beautiful and precious, but you had nothing to compare this to then, because when you are very young you haven't separated from beauty. You are just you. Think of a three-year-old little girl wearing a pretty dress, holding the skirt out, twirling around, singing "la, la, la" for no one or no reason in particular ... that little girl *knows* she is precious. She knows it in her soul. She was born knowing. But there is no consciousness for beauty at this age, because we don't associate with it, because there is been no separation from it. But as we experience more of life we begin to create meanings from what people say, from the expressions on their faces, about who we must be to have that happen "to" us. And over time, every single human creates beliefs in their own deficiency. You begin to believe, at a very young age, that you have to do certain things or be a certain way to be loved or look beautiful. Yet as a little girl, all you had to do to be loved was exist. You didn't have to *do* anything. Because at a very young age, you simply embodied beauty and you still "knew" you are beautiful.

All girls lose the "knowing" at different ages, but we lose it, and I believe that most women spend their whole lives trying to feel like this again — only they often choose mechanisms that hurt their health in the process. Many women use too much food, or food deprivation, or too much alcohol, or cigarettes or other drugs, or shopping and spending beyond their means, or brief, sometimes unsafe, intimate encounters trying to prove to themselves and others, trying to prove something they know in their soul is true: that they are beautiful and therefore, lovable.

But most of you reading this book will still be living in the haze of forgetfulness. So let this book reach the depths of your soul and awaken you to remember what you have known in your heart all along: that you are so precious and so very beautiful. While you are reading this book and also beyond this time, I want you to spend at least five minutes each day recognizing all that you contribute to this world, just by being who you are. And let that recognition light a flame inside you that with each day grows stronger and brighter from the kindness you show yourself through your lifestyle choices, including how you feed yourself, and your thoughts. And may that light guide you home to the radiance that you are.

HEARTBREAK

One of the scenarios that can lead a woman to lose her belief in her beauty is if someone she loves, usually a male, "leaves" her, or ends a relationship. Most females make it all about them, whether it was Dad who left, or a significant other who ended a relationship. They start to believe that if only they were prettier or smarter, depending on what she perceives he values, then he wouldn't have left and he would still love her. But that is not true. He left because of him. But we make it about us, and then live with the false belief that if only we were something that we now perceive we are not, then maybe we could have avoided this emotional pain.

But please reconsider what you believe about yourself with regard to men. Heartbreak is not the end of the world, even though at the time you may feel like it is. Having thrived — notice that I wrote "thrived", rather than "survived" — through a few heartbreaks myself, I offer you this: people come into our lives for a reason, and every soul who enters is a blessing. We may not see or know that at the time, but even in challenging circumstances or relationships there is an opportunity to learn more about ourselves and grow. Sometimes intimate relationships or even friendships can run their course. What once served you and/or the other person may no longer do so.

There may come a time when we need to let go with love, dignity, kindness, and respect, all the while being grateful for the joy and lessons that have blessed our lives through that person.

I say it again: "the bigger the wound, the greater the gift". When you start to deeply appreciate that life doesn't actually happen *to* you, but instead life happens *for* you, you begin to see and experience the gifts of what for you at the time may have been the toughest time in your life. Once you transform emotional pain into a great gift, without which you can see that you wouldn't be you or where you are today, whether you like where you are today or not, the next stage of growth follows. Dr Donny Epstein beautifully describes this as when "you start happening for life". When you start happening for life, you have taken the pain, transformed it into gifts, and now share that. You pass on what you have learnt, and the transformation of someone else's pain into gifts begins — a ripple effect is generated when you share your journey. It is part of how we contribute. It is part of how we learn and grow. It is part of how we return to the knowing deep in our heart, that life is precious, that we are very precious, and that we need to treat others and ourselves accordingly.

Judgment is no fun, for the judger or the person being judged. You don't need to stay connected to someone you feel is judging you. Consider, however, that when we feel judged it is usually because we have been busy judging others, although we may not be able to see that at the time. If you feel judged, explore where *you* judge. It is important to become aware of this. Judgment is detrimental to our health, and judging or being judged can lead us to feel that we have lost our shine.

I believe that to be a responsible adult we need to take responsibility for our physical health. We need to eat our vegetables and move our bodies. I also believe that, as adults, we need to take responsibility for our emotions. We need to take responsibility for how we show up for others, and we also need to own the meanings we create from interacting with others. We have to own it when someone "triggers" us, when they prod that bruise that was created in the past, often a long time before they came into our life. When we don't take responsibility for our emotions, not only can it affect our perception of our own self-worth, but it can also affect how others feel about themselves.

Once I was sitting in an audience, listening to a speaker, whom I found engaging and passionate; I was interested to hear what he had to say. After a while,

I could hear others around me start murmuring, "He thinks he's better than us." They were sitting in judgment of him for being "better than them", which is a perception. However, think about this. For someone to come across as "better than them", the person doing the viewing has to believe they are not enough. Or not good enough. Or not as good as the person speaking. The presenter had touched on their sore point of "I'm not good enough", but they couldn't see it or acknowledge it, nor could they get the gift from that perception and transform the pain from the past. They missed the opportunity because they remained stuck in the judgment. If they felt "worthy" themselves, they would never have perceived him as better than them in the first place. It is the getting stuck in the perception that prevents growth, not the perception itself.

There are flipsides to this, too. If the people who felt the speaker was "better than them" had actually been authentic and approached the speaker, and said, "You know what? You come across as though you think you are better than us", it would give the speaker the option to check in with himself and see if that rings true so he can learn and grow. And if he is a responsible adult and does not take offence at their comments, he has the opportunity to enquire with those "judging" him about what might be happening in their own lives for them to perceive him this way — that they feel they are "less than" him.

And — and this so important — if someone is coming across as "better than them", then those judging need to enquire within themselves about why that person would feel he has to show up as "better than" other people. They would then catch a glimpse of his wound and be able to bring empathy to their connection; judgment would disappear.

Judgment doesn't light anyone up. Everyone has reasons about why they are the way they are; plus you bring your version of the world to every interaction you have. Please always remember that everyone has a story. Bring empathy and/or enquiry to each interaction, and let judgment go.

FEMININITY

There is a trend in the world for women to behave in more masculine ways, while men are embodying more feminine ways. For a woman to feel or perceive her own sparkle and beauty, she often needs to reconnect to her femininity, and restorative practices and feminine rituals can assist with this.

Feminine essence and masculine essence are polar opposites. The majority of women have a feminine essence at their core; however, we have both feminine and masculine traits. Masculine energy is focused, solution-oriented, driven, and directed. It has a strong backbone. Conversely, like the ocean, the native state of the feminine is to flow with great power but no single direction. The masculine builds canals, dams, and boats to get from point A to point B, but the feminine moves in many directions at once. The masculine chooses a single goal and moves in that direction. Like a ship cutting through a vast ocean, the masculine decides on a course and navigates toward a defined destination, while feminine energy itself is undirected but immense, like the wind and deep currents of the ocean, ever-changing, beautiful, destructive, and the source of life.

Anytime you force yourself, or someone else knowingly or unknowingly drives you, to be more like a ship than an ocean, you are negating your feminine energy. Any time your man talks to you and expects you to analyse your mood and situation to the point of being able to "fix" it, he is talking "masculine" with you. You can do this — you may even be better at it than he is — but it won't make you a happy woman.

A happy woman is a woman relaxed in her body and heart: powerful, unpredictable, deep, potentially wild and destructive, or calm and serene, but always full of life, surrendered to and moved by the great force of her oceanic heart. Women do not become "free" by analysing themselves. They become free by surrendering to love. Not anyone else's love. *Their* love. They become free by surrendering to the immense flow of love that is native to their core, and by allowing their lives to be moved by this force. It may involve moments of analysis, but primarily it involves deep trust.

The feminine purpose is the flow of love in relationships (intimate, family, and friendships). The masculine priority is purpose and direction, but for many men and women today, they have lost touch with what they want and what lights them up, or they believe they can't have it or don't deserve it. If you want more love, bring more love to every situation you encounter. It sounds counter-intuitive but, whatever you want more of, share it with others. And then watch your love and connections, as well as your femininity, shine.

TRANSITION FROM SUPERFICIAL SHINE TO DEEP RADIANCE

When it comes to understandings and insights about feminine energy and radiance, no one expresses it better than that incredible teacher, David Deida, author of many books, including *The Way of the Superior Man*. The following is paraphrased from a piece of his work I read many years ago that has fostered my own deeper considerations about aging and radiance across a lifetime.

For many reasons, from biological to spiritual, masculine energy tends to be more sexually attracted to younger women rather than older women. Walking down the beach or street, a man's head is more likely to turn for a 20-year-old woman than a 60-year-old one. This is quite natural.

But feminine energy is deeper than this. Youthful sexual attractiveness is a temporary aspect of a much deeper and more fundamental quality of feminine energy: radiance. Feminine radiance is not only the flush of a woman's cheeks or the glow of her skin, it is the shine of her life force itself. A woman's true radiance reveals the degree to which she is open, trusting, connected, and loving. Her capacity to love, in turn, allows her body to be moved by the power of life force itself. Herein lies the true nature of feminine radiance and power, far beyond the simple sexiness of a naïve young woman.

When a woman is young, her body more easily conducts life force, and so she generally appears more radiant than an older woman. But even among young women, there are those who appear to be pretty just on the outside, and those whose beauty seems to spring from their depths. As a woman ages, through the processes you now understand, her skin may start to lose its youthful capacity to conduct life force. What remains obvious is her feminine radiance and depth.

In fact, as Deida says, it is this "deep beauty that the masculine finds most attractive, even in young women. There is a difference between a man's knee-jerk response to a cute babe and the open-hearted awe and mindless swoon he feels in the company of a woman who moves, breathes, smiles, and shines radiant feminine energy like a goddess." This deep feminine beauty or radiance need not be diminished by age. Rather, it can be magnified, deepened, and glorified.

If a man is disconnected from his deep masculine core of purpose and consciousness, then he will also be disconnected from a woman's depth. He will only see skin-deep, and he will be attracted to the superficial display of a woman's radiance, which often disappears with the passing of youth. He may inadvertently dishonour the true and deep forms of feminine radiance and so contribute to the social cult of youth, where women try to look and behave younger than they truly are, denying the power and radiance springing from their depths.

The natural sexiness of a young woman will always give the masculine energy. And a man need never deny this. It is part of being masculine. But the awesome beauty and radiant ease of a deep woman can stop a man's mind and widen his heart in the mystery of feminine grace, all in an instant, with a single gaze or touch, regardless of her body's age.

ESSENCES OF BEAUTY

I have noticed that people who have confronted their fears and pain and have applied the healing balm of tender care and love, seem to be rewarded with a particular kind of beauty, one that appears on the face as the radiance of wisdom, love, and peace.

For me, there are essences of beauty. One of them is truth. A beautiful face is an honest face. Not only does it reflect, to some extent, whatever is going on inside, but it also reveals a person who is genuinely coping with whatever she may be experiencing. A person who is in touch with her feelings and seeks the assistance and care she needs does not remain in an emotionally challenged state for long. She has compassion for herself, she seeks help and support when she needs it, and she wants the same for others. Be honest with others, but also with yourself. We often pride ourselves on being honest with others but won't acknowledge that the way we might be eating, drinking, and/or thinking is not serving our health.

Other essences of beauty for me include laughter, patience, generosity, kindness and love. One of the first traits we seek in another person's face is the capacity to love. As humans, we sense when a face radiates love; it reveals a person's intention and beautiful heart, although we may not mentally process this at the time of meeting. Radiate love. It will give so much to others and it will come beaming back to you.

Uniqueness is another essence of beauty for me. Through our teenage years, it is engrained in our psyche that we need to fit in and be like everyone else to be accepted, and therefore loved. But please always remember that who you are is your contribution to the world. And the world would not be the same without you. The world needs you and wants you to recognize all you contribute just by being who you are.

When I asked a friend what her essences of beauty are she said, "A smile and kind virtues. Without proper nutrition skin can be dull, but without kind virtues people lose their gloss." I loved it so much that I had to share. Smile and be kind. It's so simple and beautiful and brings love to the lives of those who encounter you. To feel good, do some good. What are your essences of beauty?

DEAR BEAUTIFUL GIRL

Dear Beautiful Girl,

Don't settle for a life that you live in the cloud of false belief that you aren't beautiful. Don't let it take until your life is about to end before you feel deep in your heart what you have always known — that you are, and have always been, beautiful. Live your life now, awake, and lit up with the knowing, impacting the lives of others with your light.

What is your word? What is the word written in gorgeous handwriting across your heart? What gift do you bring to every situation when you really show up? Name it. Is it "fun", "kindness", "joker", or "quiet observer who then shares her golden insights" (more than one word, I know!)? Or is it "magician", "angel", "wonder", "fabulousness", or "optimist"? Never underestimate the power you bring, the difference you make, and the gift you are to this world.

Never stop believing. Never stop believing in your own radiance, even if you feel others have urged you to dim your own light. You don't stop believing in the sun when the moon comes out. You don't stop believing in the moon when the clouds pass over her face. You may have a moment when you judge yourself harshly. You may have days or — hopefully not — weeks when you feel anything but beautiful. But never stop believing in your beauty, even if it momentarily disappears from your own view, because of choices you have made. You are not your behaviour. You need to take responsibility for your behaviour, but you are not it. We usually behave poorly when we perceive (notice that I say "perceive") that we have lost, or may lose, love or acceptance, or if we perceive we have failed. But there is no failure. It's all just feedback.

Be just like the sun that shines its light upon the world. Remember that you, too, light up the world with your very presence. Beauty is a light in your heart, and it doesn't just light up your own gorgeous face; it lights up the whole world. For when we let our own light shine, we give others permission to do the same. Open your eyes wide — I mean that literally — and see the wonder in the world. Open your eyes wide, knowing that there is wonder in your heart, and marvel at the wonder that you are.

Don't ask what the world needs.
Ask what makes you come alive, and go do it.
Because what the world needs is people who have
come alive.

Howard Thurman

Chapter 11
Beautiful Solutions:
for body, mind and soul

I t is always tempting when reading a book with a chapter title like this one to jump straight to the solutions, especially when you have an issue that you want resolved as soon as possible! If you think that you don't have time to read the whole book, and you just want to cut to the chase and get answers, and then put those answers into action and get your results, well, please consider this ...

If you have come to this chapter first, I cannot encourage you enough to return to the beginning of this book and read it from cover to cover. Science suggests, and I am certainly convinced from working with people for 15 years, that it helps you taking action when you know *why* you need to change something, and that knowing why can lead to a commitment to change. For, when the why is strong enough, change is a natural follow-through. If the solutions offered here were simply a list of instructions, then this section could make up the whole book. But if I don't show you *why* I am suggesting you change the way you eat, drink, move, think, believe, or perceive to get the beauty outcomes you seek, the "solutions" will only be additions to your to-do list that you may, or may not, do for two weeks, two months, or two years. Either way, before long you will return to how you have always done things, frustrated by not getting the transformations you seek.

For example, without your knowing why, I might ask you to focus on your breathing every day for the next six weeks. You might do this for a brief period, but as soon as you get beyond busy you will feel like you don't have time and the breathing sessions will cease. And with the subsequent elevated stress hormones that will most likely return without the focus on your breathing, all of the "non-vital" processes, which include the strength of your nails, the gloss of your hair, and the aliveness of your skin, are compromised. Soaring stress hormones cause your body to believe that the best use of its resources, including nutrients and blood flow, is to put them toward saving your life, not sprucing up your exterior. To that end, you need to know *why* I make the following suggestions.

Secondly, there are suggestions and solutions scattered throughout each chapter that won't necessarily be repeated here. Thirdly, I believe that you are more likely to take action and care for yourself when a particular section of this book speaks directly to you. When that happens, when you feel like I have read your diary or caught a glimpse of your life, or perhaps you got goose bumps, laughed, or cried, then you are far more compelled to act than if you simply read my recommendations below.

I begin with a set of suggestions designed to help your biochemistry switch from stress to calm. I also want to remind you at this stage in your beauty journey to please spend some time in solitude, with a journal by your side if that appeals, exploring what may have bubbled to the surface for you while reading the Beautiful Insights chapter, in particular. Once you catch a glimpse of where your false belief about a deficiency in your beauty originated, the immense power to change your whole life is in your hands; change naturally flows from this space.

Don't go into a zone of being overwhelmed when approaching changes you would like to make or changes you can see that you need to make. If you go into a sense of being overwhelmed, pay close attention, as this is likely a pattern you run regularly in life. Explore this if that is the case, because a sense of being overwhelmed is stressful for the body and the mind, as well as for the people around you. Remember, ordinary things consistently done produce extraordinary results.

Because there are solutions peppered throughout

each chapter, this chapter contains additional ideas for each area we have covered, adding to the base knowledge offered in each section. The first block of solutions, however, are general concepts that encourage what I call restorative practices. Everyone can benefit from them, whatever your individual situation. I go into detail about these in my book *Rushing Woman's Syndrome*, as well as in my 30-day coaching course called the *Rushing Woman's Syndrome Quick Start Course* (www.drlibby.com/changeyourlife) and the *Condition the Calm Advanced Course*. Restorative practices are critical for you to live from the green zone, with the parasympathetic nervous system (PNS) activated. Living from here allows the vital rest, digest, and repair work to take place inside your body, enhancing both your inner health and your outer radiance.

LAYING THE RESTORATIVE FOUNDATION

Restorative Eating

It is difficult to be kind, compassionate, and patient with others when you fill yourself with stimulants, such as too much caffeine, refined sugars, and artificial ingredients, and eat a highly processed diet virtually devoid of nutrients. I believe that if each individual were to embrace compassion, kindness, and patience, there would not be human violence in the world. But if humans fill themselves with too much caffeine, alcohol, and "dead" food, it makes it much harder for them biochemically to consistently access these gentle emotional states. A real food diet also allows you to explore your emotional landscape with clarity, and free yourself from patterns that no longer serve you.

Food becomes part of you, and the nutrients from food drive every chemical reaction inside of you. Choose real food that nourishes you, and watch your physical, as well as your emotional, health shine.

- Eat real food
    - o Nature gets it right
    - o human intervention does not

- Un-process your diet ... zigzag if you need to
    - o eat food the way it comes in Nature as often as you can
    - o relax on certain days of the week, if you want to
    - o when you are in control of your food, you "zig" and eat nourishing food; when you are at someone else's house for dinner, for example, you eat what they serve and you "zag" — that way you still get to socialize without compromising your health

- Double the amount of green plant foods you currently eat

    o add a green smoothie for breakfast or for a snack

    o take nutrient-dense leftovers for lunch instead of buying a sandwich that will likely only have a token amount of greens on it

    o use the *Real Food Chef* cookbook, which is designed to help you amp up your greens, and/or *The Real Food Chef Video Tutorial System*, where chef Cynthia Louise and I enter your kitchen to explain why and how to eat real food — it's such a fun way to learn

- Cut out, or significantly limit, caffeine, as caffeine drives the body to make adrenalin, which interferes with calm

    o take a break from coffee, black tea, and caffeinated soft drinks (soda) for four weeks

    o after that, if you want to bring it back, drink caffeinated beverages only when you go out for breakfast or perhaps on the weekends — remember, it is what you do every day that impacts your health, not what you do sometimes: your rituals create your life

o reducing caffeine intake is crucial for most women today, as adrenalin levels are usually already high, and caffeine prompts additional adrenalin production, which simply adds to your body's perception that your life is in danger

o still go to your favourite café, but instead choose green tea (which is lower in caffeine than black tea, plus it contains theanine, which buffers the effect of caffeine), herbal tea, dandelion tea (made like a latte), or occasionally order a decaf coffee (make sure it is Swiss Water filtered to limit your consumption of the usual chemicals used to decaffeinate coffee beans — most cafés have the Swiss Water filtered decaf these days); even better, order a green juice

- Cut out or significantly limit alcohol
  o get honest with yourself about how

alcohol affects you and those around you

- o if you drink it every day, it stops being special

- o drink only on special occasions

- o if you drink every day, you are drinking too much

- o if you consume more than 200 millilitres of wine a day and have less than two alcohol-free days per week, scientific research suggests you are damaging your health and increasing your risk of certain diseases, breast cancer in particular

- o swap alcohol for sparkling water with fresh lemon or lime

- o if you want to keep drinking, swap wine for gin or vodka, less alcohol (you tend to have one standard drink instead of three standard drinks per glass), less sugar, no preservatives — all liver loaders — or, better still, choose sparkling water with fresh lemon or lime for four weeks

- • follow the digestive system strategies outlined later in this chapter to maximize nourishment

Restorative Movement

If you are sympathetic nervous system (SNS) dominant from the way you live your life, adding more factors to your world that promote SNS dominance will not solve your rush. Remember, you often resist the most what you need the most. I witness this in my work with people every week of my life. If you are currently into loads of cardio, you may tell me that yoga will "bore you to tears". I call cardio "yang" exercise, and I describe some forms of yoga as "yin". Most women need to incorporate more yin movement into their lifestyle on a regular basis. I also encourage women to do some form of regular resistance training, whether that be using weights or simply using their own body weight, as happens in yoga.

Yin movement includes:

- Qigong

  o a delicious way to start the day

- Restorative yoga

  o if there is one form of movement that is deeply nourishing and replenishing for our nervous system, this is it — it truly lives up to its name — and the poses are simple to learn and easy to incorporate into your daily life (see more details later in this chapter)

  o it is particularly beneficial for those who identified with the pituitary depletion, the adrenal depletion, or the thyroid depletion health pictures

- o it is also outstanding at regulating the menstrual cycle and fertility

- o it is the most divine, feminine, restorative movement I have discovered

- Meditation
  - o the stillness that comes from regular meditation is in itself a journey and a reward

  - o if your mind is super-busy, find a CD you like that can guide you — it can help to have someone talking or asking you to imagine things for a period of time when the meditation first starts: once the mind is quieter, you will be able to embody the stillness on offer (you are welcome to try the hard-copy or downloadable *Restorative Calm* guided visualization I have created; and more resources are available at: www.drlibby. com/bioresources)

  - o remember, meditation takes practice

  - o we understand that we need to train the body: you can't run a marathon without any training, you have to work up to the distance with practice runs — the mind is the same, it takes practice to train it

o the following is a piece written by a lady who had resisted meditation but persevered with it:

> *"Today I had my usual pang of anxiety about the future and getting sick, being in an accident, losing someone who is close to me (my mind is incessant; it never stops), but then something amazing happened. I just let myself fall into the feelings and the whole thing opened up. I had read about this before but never experienced it. I felt like the entire night sky, filled with stars, was inside me. It was really amazing being able to witness a moment of terror and pain transform into something calming and expansive."*

o feel your feelings: part of growing up is learning that your feelings will not destroy you — they are just feelings, and they too shall pass.

o make it your own: maybe your meditation is during savasana on the yoga mat, maybe it is five minutes sitting cross-legged in a sunny spot in your home, maybe it is in done with a CD guiding you through; it is easier to integrate meditation into your life when you find a way to own it — try many methods, and stick with what moves you

- Daily gratitudes
  - when you are grateful you cannot be stressed — they have the opposite biochemistry and, in the split second when you are feeling one of these, you cannot feel the other

  - say out loud or write down, each day at least three things for which you are grateful (I have given you many examples throughout this book, if you don't know where to start)

  - it can be gorgeous to keep a journal to capture your gratitudes and any other murmurings that bubble to the surface while you are in this space — insight often comes this way, and we get clarity about something that we may feel confused about

- Incorporate some form of yin movement into your week. Ideally, practise at least three times per week. Better yet, you can set up a daily ritual, even if it is simply 20 long, slow breaths. Or it may mean starting out with a once a week session of yoga or some online qigong classes. Yin begets yin! Before you know it, you will be expanding your practice.

- If you insist on continuing to cardio it up every day, start your day with a yin ritual such as qigong, or be sure to have some yin days each week.

Restorative Sleep

As discussed earlier, there are a few things I link to amazing health. They include optimal nutrition, of course, fresh air, diaphragmatic breathing, living from the green zone, movement, love, gratitude, and great sleep. Sleep affects our physical and mental health enormously. Sleep is often the only time our PNS can dominate, and I suspect that for many women who don't sleep well or long enough it isn't even happening overnight. It is vital that you schedule maximum sleep time for yourself if you want to start feeling bliss from the inside out. Restorative sleep is critical to every level of our health. Of course, if you have little ones who need you during the night, support yourself to sleep when you can, and remember to breathe, and remind yourself that they are little for such a short time.

If you do not sleep well, or you do not feel restored after sleep, apply any (or all!) of the strategies below. The overall concept here is to do whatever it takes to get you to stop churning out adrenalin so that your inner health is optimal and your outer beauty can shine.

- Omit all sources of caffeine for eight weeks
  - that includes soft drinks and chocolate, as well as the obvious sources, tea and coffee
  - wean off caffeine if you currently have more than two caffeinated drinks per day, by having a green tea daily for three days and then omit it
  - after eight weeks, if it has helped your sleep, choose whether to bring it back or not
- Omit alcohol
  - you may feel like it helps you fall asleep, but it tends to disturb most people's sleep patterns during the night, as it prevents you from going into the restorative, deep REM sleep
- Do not sit in bright light for two hours before you want to go to bed
- Get up at the same time each morning, and expose your eyes to sunlight — light destroys your sleep hormone melatonin and allows your happy, calm, content hormone, sero-tonin, to surge
- Avoid doing work for a minimum of two hours before bed

- Don't use backlit devices, such as laptops, phones, or tablets for a minimum of one hour, preferably two hours, before bed, and *do not take them to bed*

- Make your bedroom a wireless-free zone: use an old-fashioned alarm clock if you need a clock to wake you, rather than sleeping with your phone beside your head, but if you want your phone in your room, leave it well away from your bed

- Go to bed before midnight, since cortisol begins to increase around 2am — an ideal time to sleep for most adults is from 10pm until 6am

- Consider the age of your bed

  o dust, mould, and sweat all accumulate in mattresses, plus beds lose their support over time: you spend one-third of your life in bed, so it is best to make it a place that brings out an "ahhh" moment of bliss when you fall into it each night (this "ahhh" moment alone is good for your health!)

  o if your bed is more than 10 years old, it is most likely not supporting you well and the waste accumulation may be affecting your health — this is particularly true if you experience allergies to dust, mould, and/or have asthma

- Schedule (and do!) 20 long, slow breaths daily — have a reminder pop up on your computer, for example, at 3pm every day

- Do restorative yoga poses daily; each evening before sleep is particularly beneficial

- Meditate and/or pray regularly

Restorative Actions

Feeling like your life has purpose and meaning is crucial to restorative actions. Contribution is key here. When you make a difference in someone else's life, your heart feels full. As the poet Rabindranath Tagore so beautifully said: "I slept and dreamt that life was joy. I awoke and saw that life was service. I acted and behold, service was joy."

- Pick up any litter you see

- Call people you may not have caught up with for ages — they will be thrilled to hear from you

- Volunteer

  o a male friend of mine who works in a more than full-time job was standing on a street corner collecting money for the City Mission, who, among many things, raise money for food to feed people: he said he does a half day for them every month — I had no idea, as he had never

mentioned it — and said it was the least
he could do because he has so much

- Bake a cake and deliver it to an aged-care
  facility, and stay a while and talk to the resi-
  dents — you will not only make their day,
  you will learn something

- Give the clothes you no longer wear to an
  organization that can use them

- Smile at others while you walk along the
  street

- Notice the colour of the sky wherever you are

- Send someone a card in the mail to let them
  know you are thinking of them

  o my amazing mum has sent me an
    envelope packed with bits and pieces
    every week of my life since I left
    home, to wherever I am in the world!
    (it is usually filled with pictures from
    magazines she has collected that she
    thinks I will like, and the births, deaths,
    and marriages from the local paper from
    my hometown) — it always makes my
    day (thanks, Mum)

- If you think of something that amuses you,
  and you think it would entertain others, tell
  them or text them — share the entertainment
  and giggles

- If you see someone looking lost, ask if you can help
- Practise random acts of kindness
- Be kind — as I love to say, kindness must come first

RADIANT LIVING

There are many different forms of yoga, and yoga means different things to different people. I find people gravitate to yoga for a wide variety of reasons. For some, it is about movement, flexibility, and strength. For others, it is a spiritual practice. For some, it is a path to stillness. Some begin because they developed a degenerative disease, such as cancer, or they see yoga as a preventative health practice. Others think it is just a cool thing to do; all of their friends are doing it. For many, whatever their reason for practising yoga, it is how they bring balance into their hectic lives. In yoga circles, they talk of the Sages' 10 Rituals of Radiant Living. I encourage you to explore each ritual for yourself, and embrace them in ways that are meaningful to you.

The Sages' 10 Rituals of Radiant Living
1. Ritual of Solitude
2. Ritual of Physicality
3. Ritual of Nourishment
4. Ritual of Abundant Knowledge

5. Ritual of Personal Reflection

6. Ritual of Early Awakening

7. Ritual of Music

8. Ritual of Spoken Word

9. Ritual of Congruent Character

10. Ritual of Simplicity

KEEPING A JOURNAL

Buy yourself a beautiful notebook that can be your journal. Capture anything you like in there. Or, if you started this book with one by your side, as I suggested, don't put it aside when you read the last page. Continue to capture anything you like. Be sure to express your gratitude as a daily ritual. If you feel like you don't have time, keep it in the living room or the kitchen — some place in your house where you will see it. Keep a pen with it or, better still, some coloured markers, and whenever you clap eyes on it, think of something for which you are grateful and write it down!

Stop, Keep, Start

Another great thing to do with a journal is to make a list with the following headings:

- Stop

- Keep

- Start

Fill each column in as you respond to the questions below with your inner health and outer beauty in mind:

- What am I going to stop doing?
- What am I going to keep doing?
- What am I going to start doing?

You can use the suggestions on these pages to give you ideas. Here is a sample:

Stop	Keep	Start
I am going to stop getting caught up in gossip, as it is exhausting.	I am going to keep eating a nourishing breakfast every day.	I am going to start walking four days out of seven for the next two weeks, starting tomorrow morning at 6am.

Stop, keep, and start plans can make change fun, manageable, and suitable for your lifestyle.

EXPLORING YOUR INNER WORLD AND EMOTIONAL LANDSCAPE

The peace you seek is within you. People mistakenly wait until their external world is quiet in order to feel peaceful. For many, their external world is rarely quiet! To help you explore your inner world, to begin your enquiry, to help you understand your subconscious reactions more, to help you lose the emotional charge from a relationship that in your head you are over, but yet your body still seems to react … try any of the following:

- network spinal analysis (NSA)
  - NSA involves gentle, precise touch to the spine that cues the brain to create new wellness-promoting strategies, developing two unique healing waves, which are associated with spontaneous release of spinal and life tensions, and the use of existing tension as fuel for spinal re-organization and enhanced wellness
  - practitioners combine their clinical assessments of spinal refinements with the patient's self-assessments of wellness and life changes
  - greater self-awareness and conscious awakening to the relationships between the body, mind, emotion, and expression of the human spirit are realized through this incredible healing work (NSA is exclusively practised by chiropractors)
- The Journey
  - created by the gifted Brandon Bays, this process, described in her book of the same name, allows you to see the world as it really is, rather than the

stories you have constructed around things: it allows you to see the beliefs that no longer serve you and allow them to effortlessly fall away — and, as you now understand, when your beliefs change, your behaviour changes, as your behaviours are the outermost expression of your beliefs

- o The Journey is a powerful healing tool simply through fostering the innate healing within you

- o it would not surprise me if one day science can show what many people already believe to be true; that cellular changes can be fostered through thought — I truly believe this to be the case

- the work of Tony Robbins

  - o Tony's book *Awaken the Giant Within* is brilliant — don't just read it, do the exercises in it

  - o Tony's live event Date With Destiny is powerful beyond measure — he is a genius: his work, also available on CDs, allows you to see and then change your limiting beliefs, along with the emotions you feel you want to avoid, and foster those you want to experience; his work,

his contribution to the world, has
forever changed the face of psychology
and helps people, no matter how
massive or relatively small their past
hurts may have been, move forward into
an empowered future

- restorative yoga
    - I personally had never experienced such
      deep stillness before restorative yoga
      became part of my life (the gracious,
      kind, and insightful Tracy Whitton was
      my first teacher of this beautiful practice,
      and I am eternally grateful to her for
      developing Stillness Through Movement
      — thank you for sharing this with the
      world, beautiful lady)

    - it consists of yoga poses, pranayama
      (extension and control of the breath),
      breath awareness exercises, and
      meditation (training the mind in
      openness and kindness) — and the
      technique helps restore the body/mind
      connection

    - Stillness Through Movement is a process
      where you learn to align with your true
      consciousness/intelligence, rather than
      the stories

- through breath and mind awareness, you are able to let go, which allows you to deeply receive the benefits of the restorative pose, bringing the body/mind back to its natural state of peace and contentment

- without this awareness, you tend to live in a permanent state of unease; when you practise in this way, you begin to align with the ease of life — your new saying might just become "Life is simple and easy!"

- the PNS is effectively activated during restorative yoga: as you now know, the PNS is responsible for balancing the body and bringing its response system back into equilibrium; restorative yoga takes the spine and nervous system out of the "flight, fight or freeze" response, relaxing and calming the adrenals

- to do this, props are used to support the body so that no strain occurs; you hold each posture anywhere from 2 minutes to 20 minutes (it is sometimes referred to as "active relaxation")

- some poses target a certain area or

gland, such as the pituitary, while others have an overall benefit; all poses create specific physiological responses, which are beneficial to health and can reduce the effects of stress-related disease — in general, restorative yoga is great for those times when one feels weak, fatigued, or stressed from day-to-day activities, or for those who find other styles of yoga too difficult

o these poses are especially beneficial for those times before, during, and after major life transitions, like the death of a loved one, change of job, pregnancy, marriage, new baby, children leaving home, or divorce; you can also practise the poses when ill or recovering from an illness or injury (it is particularly beneficial for people experiencing adrenal fatigue), or simply incorporate them into your life on a daily or weekly basis

o it is great for rebalancing hormones in women who have PMS, girls with a physically or emotionally challenging puberty, and during menstruation or menopause

○ what is also exceptional about restorative yoga is that it doesn't matter whether you have never experienced yoga before or have been practising for 30 years — it is accessible, blissful, powerful, and transformational, whatever your level of experience (I personally LOVE it!)

THE SERENITY PRAYER

Don't worry about something until it is a problem. If it becomes a problem, then you can face it; worrying about something that may never happen only serves to hurt you. The ripple effect of a worry can very slowly and subtly change your mood, your metabolism, your face, and your posture. And it is the chemical signals of your body that are driving this. The beautiful, old piece of wisdom called "The Serenity Prayer" is useful to remember and act on, especially if you are a worrier:

God, grant me the serenity to accept the things
I cannot change,
Courage to change the things I can,
And the wisdom to know the difference.

And as Geneen Roth so eloquently says: "Every time you stop fighting with the way things are, you return to yourself, to Heaven on Earth. Can you stop fighting today? Can you give yourself that much of Heaven?" Grace is accepting what is instead of resenting what isn't. There is great freedom and a slice of Heaven in acceptance.

STRATEGIES TO ASSIST YOU CHAPTER-BY-CHAPTER

BEAUTIFUL FOODS, BEAUTIFUL NUTRIENTS, AND BEAUTIFUL HYDRATION

These three chapters contain specific advice about how to amp up the nutrient density of your meals and snacks, as well as the specific role certain nutrients and water play in your inner health and outer beauty. Please revisit these chapters and make notes about where you want to focus to get the outcomes you seek. The basis of your plan needs to be a focus not on eating less of anything, but a focus on eating more — more real food! Amp up your greens, now that you understand why this is critical to your beauty.

Furthermore, no amount of topical nutrients can make up for a lousy diet, nor can supplements mask the potentially long-term aging and detrimental effects of a poor diet. A focus on real food must come first. Use the *Real Food Chef* cookbook, as it is a whole cooking system born from the desire to inspire you to eat low human-intervention food — real food the way it comes in Nature. Filled with delicious, nourishing recipes, beautiful images, quotes to inspire, and food education, the *Real Food Chef* is designed to enhance your quality of life and give you more energy to live the life you love.

We eat, on average, 35 times each week, and these eating occasions supply the cells of your body with nutrients to give you optimal health, energy, and vitality. If right now seven out of your 35 meals and snacks would get the *Real Food Chef* tick of approval, then aim to include one new real food meal and/or snack per week for the next two months — just one extra per week — and in eight tiny weeks you will be at 15 out of 35 meals getting the *Real Food Chef* tick; and you will have literally doubled the amount of nutrients going into your body. Don't make the transition to more real food bigger in your mind than it actually is. Do what you can to support your inner health and outer beauty, and discover how real food can revolutionize how you feel and appear. And be sure to drink plenty of clean water!

Not-So-Beautiful Stress Hormones

How high your level of stress is and how you feel your body copes with it will influence the steps you take. The Restorative Foundation section of solutions is general, although I can confidently say that virtually everyone will benefit from applying them.

The herbs used for adrenal support are beautiful;

however, it is best to check with a qualified medical herbalist to find out about herbs that will meet your specific needs. I have made comments beside most of the herbs about their applications.

If you have identified that you are adrenally fatigued and beyond exhausted on a daily basis, your adrenal support is listed separately, and restorative yoga would be extra wonderful for you.

Solutions for Adrenal Support

✓ Schedule and commit to regular diaphragmatic breathing exercises. It can literally change your life. And I do not say that lightly.

✓ Practise yoga, Pilates, t'ai chi, or qigong a minimum of twice a week for four weeks. Develop a daily practice for outstanding results.

✓ Spend five minutes, daily, focusing on and giving voice to all the aspects of your life for which you are grateful — you can't be stressed when you feel grateful.

✓ With the guidance of a herbalist, take some adrenal support herbs. I am not associated with any brands of herbs, but when I have good reason to favour one I will mention it. When it comes to herbs, nothing compares to Mediherb, an Australian-based company (whose products are available internationally) with the highest of standards. We use liquid tinctures and the tablet combinations in my practice. The majority of these adrenal herbs are adaptogens, meaning they help the body adapt to stress by fine-tuning the stress response. They include:

- o withania, for the worriers

- o rhodiola, for the drama queens, or occasionally for the worriers

- o Siberian ginseng, for the fatigued feminine

- o panex ginseng, for the utterly fatigued

- o licorice, especially if your blood pressure is on the low end of normal

- o rehmannia, if you feel depleted but your blood pressure is the higher end of normal

- o dandelion leaves, especially if you retain fluid.

✓ The adrenals also love vitamin B and vitamin C, and for adrenal support I usually supplement both; the Bs in the form of a multivitamin (I highly rate USANA's Multi Essentials, proven scientifically to have the best absorption of any multi available; plus it has great results clinically for people) or a straight B complex, plus 4–5 grams per day of vitamin C, preferably in powdered form with added calcium and magnesium. If you are on an oral contraceptive pill, stick to 2 grams of vitamin C per day.

✓ Just as important, if not the *most* important aspect of supporting adrenal function for a balanced and appropriate stress hormone response, is the application of the emotional health strategies (explored in the Beautiful Insights chapter, as well as in my *Rushing Woman's Syndrome* book and courses) and diaphragmatic breathing.

Adrenal Fatigue Supplementation

For people with deep, deep fatigue, I often use an herbal tonic that contains:

✓ Panex ginseng or Siberian ginseng

✓ licorice

✓ dandelion leaves

✓ astragalus

✓ one other herb, depending on what else is going on for the individual (a liver herb or a reproductive herb are typical).

I will also sometimes use a range of supplements from the United States created by Dr James Wilson specifically for adrenal fatigue. I have had countless clients take this range of supplements for three months and had their energy and vitality return to great levels.

The Restorative Power of Real Food

Even though I often recommend good-quality supplements of herbs and/or nutrients for adrenal fatigue, and other health conditions, never underestimate the healing and restorative power of food the way it comes in Nature. As I have reminded you numerous times throughout this book, taking supplements is not a reason to eat a poor-quality, low-nutrient diet. I simply recommend high-quality supplements where appropriate, and especially to assist in the restoration of health.

Peri- and Postmenopause

If you are peri- or postmenopausal, I can't encourage you enough to address adrenal health and liver health, as these two systems, as well as the overall balance of your nervous system, tend to make all the difference to your menopause symptoms.

BEAUTIFUL SEX HORMONES

Menstrual Cycle Challenges

✓ If you have any type of menstrual cycle or reproductive system challenge, take a four-week break from alcohol or, better still, take a break from it for two menstrual cycles. You will see your premenstrual syndrome (PMS) significantly decrease.

✓ If this solution is "impossible", decrease alcohol intake to two nights a week, and ensure you drink less than half a bottle of wine. It is time to get honest about how alcohol may affect you.

✓ Coffee can be another big-ticket item when it comes to PMS, via liver congestion. Consider swapping coffee for green tea for four weeks, or preferably two menstrual cycles, and see how you feel.

✓ Take a four-week strict break from all dairy products.

Oestrogen Dominance

For oestrogen dominance, which can be assessed with a saliva test or a blood test measuring the different types of oestrogen and progesterone (as a start), or if you relate strongly to what is described in the oestrogen dominance symptom section:

✓ Extracts of broccoli or broccoli sprouts. I am all for getting what we need from our food, but, when oestrogen is dominant, taking a concentrated form of what broccoli has to offer can make a big difference. I love MH Enhance P2 Detox Powder.

✓ For the low progesterone that usually accompanies oestrogen dominance, then restorative practices — the breathing work in particular — as well as stress hormone reduction are key to ensuring ovulation and good progesterone production from the corpus luteum.

✓ For PMS, the following table may be useful. You may experience one or a number of different PMS patterns at once. This is simply a guide to get you started exploring where your biochemistry may need support.

The different types of PMS: the mechanisms involved, and the potential treatments.			
	Symptoms	Mechanism	Potential treatment
PMS-1	Anxiety Nervous tension Irritability Mood swings Insomnia	Elevated oestrogen Low progesterone High cortisol	Vitex Dong quai Vitamin B P2 Detox Real food
PMS-2	Water and sodium retention Abdominal bloating Weight gain Breast tenderness	Elevated aldosterone (fluid) Low dopamine	Dandelion leaves P2 Detox Vitamin B Vitex Rhodiola Real food

	Symptoms	Mechanism	Potential treatment
PMS-3	Craving sweets Increased appetite Can't resist refined sugar, followed by palpitations and fatigue Dizziness, shakiness, headache	Low magnesium Deficiency of prostaglandin PGE_1 (an anti-inflammatory substance) Elevated insulin	Magnesium Essential fats (UDO's oil, or a flax and evening primrose oil combination) Cinnamon Real food
PMS-4	Period pain and clots	Elevated prostaglandin PGE_2 (pro-inflammatory; increases inflammation in the body) Deficiency of anti-inflammatory substances Possible magnesium deficiency	Bupleurum if clots Dong quai Magnesium P2 Detox Essential fats — fish oil, or flax oil if vegetarian Dairy free diet trial; sometimes it is also necessary to eliminate gluten Real food

Endometriosis

o Dairy-free diet trial strictly for two menstrual cycles.

- o No coffee for two menstrual cycles.

- o No alcohol for two menstrual cycles.

- o No refined sugar for two menstrual cycles.

- o Amp up the plant content of your diet for two menstrual cycles.

- o Anti-inflammatory and hormone balancing fats, such as flax oil and evening primrose oil as a food-based liquid.

- o Liver support: P2 Detox Powder.

- o Herbs: typically dong quai and bupleurum.

Polycystic Ovarian Syndrome (PCOS)

- ✓ Must start with cortisol management/adrenal solutions.

- ✓ Restorative practices are key to regaining hormonal balance.

- ✓ The imbalance between oestrogen and progesterone needs to be addressed, as does what are often elevated androgens (but the cortisol and stress management is the first step, as the other factors respond faster and come into balance in less time when cortisol is addressed first).

✓ Ensure good communication between the pituitary and the ovaries, which the herb vitex can support.

Menopause Strategies

✓ For hot flashes, consider whether the heat is coming from low oestrogen, liver/gallbladder congestion, or both.

- For low oestrogen, black cohosh and sage can be useful.

- For the liver/gallbladder, globe artichoke, St Mary's thistle, bupleurum, and schisandra are excellent.

✓ Please note that if you decide to supplement hormonal activity in *any* way — whether it be through conventional medicine, bioidentical hormones, or herbally — I cannot encourage you enough to support your liver detox pathways at the same time (more on that below). Whatever the source of the hormones, you must be able to detoxify them and excrete them once they have done their job in your body.

✓ For adrenal support, rhodiola, Siberian ginseng, and withania can be appropriate; you may like to consult with a medical herbalist for a specific prescription to meet your individual needs.

✓ For low blood pressure, licorice is excellent.

✓ Magnesium for nervous system support and relaxation.

For all of the sex hormone challenges, focus, too, on the gifts of your feminine essence, explored in the Beautiful Insights chapter.

BEAUTIFUL THYROID HORMONES

✓ Go on a gluten-free diet trial for a minimum of four weeks. Some people will do better committing to this for a minimum of three months so that they begin to feel an improved level of wellness or improvements in their blood work.

✓ If you *love* dairy products and the idea of going without cheese makes you wonder if you could, then do it! Remember, it is often what we love to eat — not just like — that can be a problem. Do a four-week dairy-free trial if this is the case for you.

✓ Support liver and gallbladder function to assist with bowel elimination. Globe artichoke can be particularly good for someone whose thyroid needs support.

✓ Refer to the advice about oestrogen dominance, as excess oestrogen can interfere with thyroid function.

✓ Adrenal support is almost essential, especially when beginning to treat the thyroid. Refer to the stress hormones solutions to refresh on adrenal support strategies.

✓ You will probably crave coffee. Please explore taking a four-week break and observe how you feel at the end of this period. Use green tea, which has a low caffeine level, instead. If that feels "impossible" and you decide to keep having coffee, please only have one and make it before 11am.

✓ If you have a diagnosed, under-active thyroid condition, and you are on synthetic medication but your symptoms are still present, explore transitioning to a different brand of medication, or whole thyroid extract, under medical supervision.

✓ See a health professional for guidance about what minerals are best suited to meet your individual needs. For example, you may need additional iodine, selenium, iron, and/or essential fats.

✓ Explore how you can change the "demands" on your time if you have an over-active thyroid.

✓ Daily restorative practices are very important for you to support your whole endocrine system.

BEAUTIFUL PITUITARY HORMONES

✓ Restorative yoga

✓ Herbs: vitex, alfalfa, ginseng family, licorice

✓ Oils: sandalwood, clary sage, massaged into the soles of your feet and/or reproductive organ areas

When the pituitary gland is at the heart of someone's problem — please understand that I am not referring to pituitary diseases — they will often have suboptimal health with a number of endocrine organs, which may include the ovaries (sex hormones), the adrenals (stress hormones), and/or the thyroid (thyroid hormones). They will also, most likely, have been living in SNS dominance for some time. When I suspect the pituitary needs support, I tend to use vitex for a woman who is menstruating and rhodiola post-menopausally. If the pituitary gland is at the heart of your situation, I recommend that you choose one of the systems referenced above and start there — many people start with the adrenals — or consult with an experienced health professional to guide you. You are welcome to reach out to my practice if that appeals. We do consultations all over the world via Skype or telephone. Or simply start supporting the pituitary by doing restorative yoga. This alone can be incredibly healing.

BEAUTIFUL DETOX

It is important for you to remember that there are numerous ways our body detoxifies, as outlined throughout the book. However, if you identify that your liver health needs to be addressed to resolve what may be ongoing skin challenges, PMS, or intense eruptions of anger, here are some solutions to support your liver detox processes.

Alcohol and Caffeine Consumption

Set yourself a time-based goal when it comes to making these changes. For example, "I will drink alcohol only on weekends for four weeks" or "I will drink coffee only when I go out for breakfast on Sundays." If you leave it open-ended when you initially make some changes, if you eat/drink in a way you said you wouldn't, you may feel like you have "ruined" it. You haven't ruined anything — you just had a [fill in the blank naming whatever you ate/drank]. If you make the initial change period time-based, you can review your changes after a period of time.

✓ Take a break from alcohol.

✓ Only drink on weekends; no alcohol during the week.

✓ Replace coffee with green or white tea (or, less often, weak, black tea), or swap all hot drinks to herbals (no caffeine).

Liver Support Herbs

Liver support herbs may be beneficial such as:
✓ St Mary's thistle, especially if alcohol is/has been a regular part of your life

- ✓ globe artichoke, especially of you have a tendency to constipation, a liver roll (fat roll under your bra), or central torso tenderness

- ✓ bupleurum, especially if there are clots in the menstrual blood

- ✓ schisandra, especially for its detox action (it also works on the adrenals)

- ✓ MH Enhance P2 Detox Powder, which is highly effective at supporting just what its name suggests — phase 2 liver detox pathways; many people do well taking this additional liver support daily regardless of what is happening with their health and/or beauty — we are exposed to more substances today than ever before that our body has to detoxify (transform) before we can excrete them.

Additional Solutions

- ✓ Transform anger into passion by giving a different meaning to a past experience; the energy of anger and passion are very similar. We get angry when we perceive that our needs aren't being met, so see anger as a sign of this.

- ✓ Drink vegetable juice or a green smoothie each morning.

- ✓ Amp up the vegetable content of your diet. Eat more real food, as it contains substances that enhance detox; plus, when you eat more real food, you subsequently eat fewer liver loaders and processed foods.

✓ Snack on seeds and nuts.

✓ Trial eating less fruit, and none after morning tea.

✓ Cut out dairy products for a four-week trial and/ or omit grains containing gluten for a four-week trial.

✓ Take an essential fatty acid supplement — a good-quality, decent dose of fish oil for reducing cholesterol, or a flax oil and evening primrose combination for hormonal imbalances.

✓ Eat high-zinc foods, such as oysters (from clean waters), or take a zinc supplement of zinc picolinate 15–30 milligrams per day — best taken at night just before bed to maximize absorption.

Remember, it is what you do every day that impacts on your health, not what you do sometimes. Just get honest with yourself. And take such good care of yourself that your quality of life is forever excellent. We only have one liver!

Beautiful Digestion

Digestion is central and essential to every process in our body, especially our beauty. It is the base on which we build. So, whether your aim is to slow down, weigh less, optimize your health and well-being, improve a challenging or diseased gut, resolve acute or chronic skin challenges, or all of the above, understanding your digestive system is a crucial step to optimal health.

Solutions

✓ Slow down! Chew your food. Swallow each mouthful before you put the next mouthful in.

✓ Include fats and/or protein with each meal, as you are likely to eat less and be satisfied with less total food for that meal, than if you simply eat carbohydrates on their own.

✓ If you overeat, decide to eat less. Reduce your portion size by one-quarter, especially in the evening if you tend to over-eat, and see how you feel. Explore your beliefs using ideas in the Beautiful Insights chapter about why you do this, or read *Accidentally Overweight*, as I explore emotional eating in great detail there.

✓ If you know you don't eat enough, and you now understand that this ages you and harms your physical and emotional well-being, explore your beliefs using ideas in the Beautiful Insights chapter about why you do this. Capture your insights in a journal, and make a decision to focus on nourishing your body, mind, and soul, rather than starving them.

✓ Wake up your stomach acid before you eat, by using lemon juice in warm water or apple cider vinegar before meals, breakfast in particular.

✓ Drink water between meals, not with meals.

✓ If efficient bowel evacuation is a particular challenge for you, reference *Accidentally Overweight* and the numerous strategies outlined there.

✓ Omit a food you feel you cannot live without for a trial period of four weeks. The first four to seven days will be the most difficult, but persevere. The results may be enormously worth it.

✓ Working with a practitioner of traditional Chinese medicine can also assist you in healing your gut.

✓ Try aloe vera juice to start your day if you have a particularly irritated gut.

✓ Eat in a calm state so that the blood flow to the digestive system is well supported. Blood is diverted to your periphery (arms and legs) when you are living on adrenalin, as your body is fuelling you to get you ready to get out of danger.

✓ Look at your food while you eat it. Do not read or watch television while you eat.

✓ If you suspect a parasite infection, the herbs black walnut and Chinese wormwood are excellent, as is oregano oil.

✓ If you suspect you have some not-so-nice gut bacteria that are fermenting your food, apply all of these strategies first to see if that helps, as often the bad guys have been able to take over because of the pH of the large intestine, and this is mostly influenced by what goes on higher up in the digestive system. If these strategies don't work, trial a probiotic supplement that contains *Bifidobacterium* species.

✓ If you suspect you are reacting to a food, strictly omit that food from your diet for a period of four weeks. If it makes no difference, bring it back. If it helps, leave it out for three months, and then try it again. Or if you are happy to go without it, then do so. If it is a food that is a rich source of nutrients — for example, gluten-containing foods tend to be a good source of B vitamins — then you will need to supplement. It will also be necessary to supplement with a mineral supplement that contains a combination of calcium, magnesium, manganese, boron, and vitamin D if you omit dairy products. This is of lesser importance if your diet is caffeine-free, plant-based, and highly alkaline. It is best to seek the guidance of a health professional if you are going to omit food(s) to get a resolution of your symptoms on a longer-term basis.

✓ Chamomile is one of the best remedies for constipation and complete evacuation. This is because it can soften the waste and help the bowel wall relax. Either drink lots of tea, or take capsules with each meal. I am a huge fan of this beautiful herb.

Colonics

Another potential remedy is one that many people have strong opinions about — colon hydrotherapy, or colonics. This process involves inserting a tube into the rectum through which warm or cool water then gently flows. This softens the hardened faecal matter allowing the large bowel to empty fully, getting rid of built-up waste that may have been there for a long time.

Colonics polarize people. Note, however, that right up until the early 1900s, colon hydrotherapy was part of general medicine, and was once accepted as a very "normal" treatment method for a host of health conditions, not just bowel issues. Seek advice from a health professional before undertaking colon hydro-therapy if it appeals to you.

BEAUTIFUL SLEEP

Please refer to the Laying the Restorative Foundation solutions above, as sleep is a critical aspect of restoration, and ideas for better, more restorative sleep are outlined there.

BEAUTIFUL POSTURE AND MOVEMENT

Explore, and incorporate into your life, movements that serve you. Remember your movement needs may change over time. Let your body give you feedback about what it needs, and do what you enjoy. Dancing may be your new beauty medicine!

Explore how one or all of the following can be incorporated into your life regularly:

- ✓ restorative movement
- ✓ functional movement
- ✓ weight-bearing movement
- ✓ stretching.

Remember, too, that how you carry yourself communicates messages to your internal body and chemistry, and also to the outside world, about how you feel about the world and yourself. While good posture used to be talked about in beauty circles, it seems to be less so these days. Become conscious of your posture. Network spinal analysis is a wonderful modality to help transform old postural and, therefore, emotional patterns.

Beautiful Skin, Hair And Nails

You now understand that beautiful skin really is an inside job. Without great food, nutrients, hydration, digestion, liver and kidney function, as well as sex hormone balance, just to name a few, it can be a challenge for skin to keep up with the load it is being asked to excrete, causing you frustration and grief in the process. For beautiful skin, start by applying the strategies for one or all of these areas. Remember that the beauty bits get compromised when stress hormones are being churned out, as non-vital processes, such as how white your teeth are, your skin sparkle, nail strength, and hair, brow, and eyelash lush factor are not deemed important to your survival when you are on red alert.

If you want to heal your skin, you have to heal your gut. Make sure you are getting optimal nourishment from your food. Pay particular attention to your intake of:

- ✓ essential fats

- ✓ vitamin C

- ✓ zinc

- ✓ vitamin E

- ✓ all antioxidants.

Skin care

When it comes to your skin care, support the functioning of this vital organ, rather than forcing the skin to behave in a way that is not natural to it. There are plenty of beautiful skin-care companies that create highly effective products without any synthetic chemicals; they allow the skin to do its work, which includes a self-regulating oil/sebum mechanism. Embrace natural skin care for the planet and for you.

ADDITIONAL BEAUTIFUL SOLUTIONS TO BEAUTY BUMPS IN THE ROAD

Here is my take on what I have seen work with some common beauty challenges.

Eyes and Around the Eyes

Dark Circles

Focus on digestion and/or liver support. Based on what you have learnt in this book and what has welled up for you, trial either a dairy-free diet or a gluten-free diet for four weeks to see if it makes a difference. I have seen both dietary trials resolve dark circles, and I don't say that lightly. Liver herbs can also be beneficial.

Dry Eyes or Floaters in Vision

Focus on liver support. Check for iron deficiency as well.

Puffy Eyes

Adrenal support is very important. Drink only water or herbal tea for two weeks and see if this makes a difference.

Thinning Outer Third of Eyebrow

You need endocrine system support, which the Laying the Restorative Foundation section above describes. Focus particularly on thyroid support. You may even like to have some thyroid tests done. However, remember that if they show up in the "normal" range they may be skewed one way, and in this case you need to treat the signs that your body is giving you, rather than the blood results.

Hair and Scalp

Brittle Hair

Support your thyroid, adrenals, essential fatty acids, and vitamin C.

Dandruff, Flaky Scalp

This can be a vitamin A deficiency, essential fatty acids deficiency, or gut dysbiosis. If you believe that for you it is more likely to be the latter, and that there are some less-than-friendly bacterial species living in your large intestine, trial a diet where you eat zero refined sugar, and eat carbs only from whole food sources, such as root vegetables. Trial this initially for four weeks, and, if you feel there is an improvement, continue for a total of three months to assess if it will resolve in this period. You might also like to add more coconut to your diet, as the lauric acid may also assist the scalp. Amp up the greens and the whole food fat in your diet as well.

Grey Hair

Head hair going grey is mostly genetic and hereditary. However, traditional Chinese medicine treats grey hair by using herbs to support the kidneys. I have only known people of Asian heritage who have used these herbs, but that is not to say they won't benefit people of non-Asian heritage. If pubic hairs start to go grey, it can be a sign that adrenal support is necessary.

Hair Loss

Support your thyroid, adrenals, sex hormone balance, and vitamin D status.

Hairy Chin, Facial Hair

This is often due to increased levels of androgens in the skin. Start with stress hormone management strategies, including the restorative practices. When facial hair has started to occur, it is very important for these girls/women to learn how to live from a calm place, not just access a calm place when they do yoga and then go back to living with adrenal-depleting intensity.

Lips and Around the Mouth

Bad Breath

Focus on resolving gut/digestion challenges.

Chapped Lips

Focus on digestive system support, and support stomach acid production, using lemon juice in warm water or apple cider vinegar.

Cracks at the Corners of the Mouth

This can be due to a vitamin B deficiency, an iron deficiency, or both.

Teeth Strength and Prevention of Cavities

Minerals such as calcium, magnesium, manganese, boron, and vitamin D all strengthen teeth. If you notice significant changes to your teeth, consider seeing a holistic dentist, focus on a refined-sugar-free, mineral-rich, alkaline diet, and offer adrenal support. Brush twice daily. Floss. Smile ☺

Nails

Dull Nails

This can indicate poor diet, poor digestion, or a folate deficiency, especially if on the OCP. Amp up your greens, along with supporting digestion.

Lined Nails — Grooves Across the Nail

Adrenal support may be needed, and restorative practices are essential.

Lined Nails — Grooves from Base to Tip

This can indicate mineral deficiency, such as calcium and magnesium. It can also indicate that the thyroid needs support.

Pale, Brittle, Withered or Weak Nails

Liver support is necessary; it can also indicate an iron deficiency. If dietary iron intake is good, have iron blood studies done to determine if a deficiency exists. If so, explore why. "Unexplained" iron deficiency can highlight digestive system challenges or celiac disease.

Peeling or Scabby Cuticles

This can be iron deficiency, essential fatty acids deficiency, or due to SNS dominance. Apply the appropriate strategy/strategies. Also try a rubbing a little coconut oil around your nail beds each evening.

Soft Nails

Make sure you are getting adequate dietary protein. If you are sure that you are, focus on digestive system support. To make keratin, a tough protein that is a major component in hard, strong nails, the body needs high-quality protein.

Spoon-Shaped Nails

This is often due to iron deficiency. May also be deficiencies in vitamin B_{12} and/or folate.

White Spots on Nails

This can indicate a zinc deficiency.

Skin

Back-ne

This follows the same process as described for acne. Quite often a sex hormone imbalance perpetuates it, arising from high levels of androgens in the skin, elevated prolactin, or an imbalance between oestrogen and progesterone. All of these situations can be tested for if the condition is ongoing or if it doesn't respond to the sex hormone balancing suggestions, including liver support. The first place I start is with stress management, due to the role cortisol plays in the conversion of other hormones to androgens, as explained in the Beautiful Sex Hormones chapter.

Body Odour

This is usually a call for additional liver support.

Bumps on Backs of Arms

This can be the result of an essential fatty acids deficiency and/or due to excess fruit consumption. If essential fatty acids are supplemented, including evening primrose oil in the mix can be helpful.

Cellulite

Liver and lymphatic support has been shown to decrease the appearance of cellulite. Rebounding is a wonderful way to stimulate the lymphatic system. Significantly limiting or omitting liver loaders has also been shown to reduce the appearance of cellulite or in some cases allows it to disappear.

Cold Sores

They are caused by the Herpes virus, so immune support is vital; consider using additional vitamin C and zinc, and some immune support herbs. Herpes only reactivates itself when you trigger it with stress, poor dietary choices, or too little sleep. Herpes is like a seed in a desert. It will stay asleep indefinitely if the signal to germinate isn't given. It is also important to minimize intake of foods that can feed viruses, such as reducing dietary exposure to the amino acid arginine. When the amino acid lysine is higher in your diet than the amino acid arginine, herpes has trouble replicating. When arginine is higher than lysine, herpes multiplies quickly. Foods high in arginine include chocolate, crustaceans, soy, and peanuts.

Cracked Elbows

This indicates an essential fatty acid deficiency and/or zinc deficiency.

Cracked Heels

This often indicates a deficiency in essential fatty acids.

Dry Skin

This may indicate an essential fatty acids deficiency, poor skin-care choice, thyroid dysfunction, poor diet, or poor digestion.

Eczema in Adults

Follow a strict dairy-free diet trial for four weeks. If that doesn't make a difference at all, bring dairy back, and omit all red foods, such as chillies, capsicums (peppers), tomatoes, strawberries, apples (red and green), for a four-week trial and see if that makes a difference. Or, if you eat more than two pieces of fruit a day, cut back to less than two, or omit fruit for a trial period of four weeks to see if that makes a difference. An evening primrose oil supplement can also be highly beneficial, as it contains an enzyme called delta-6-desaturase, which allows fat to be incorporated into the skin, keeping it moist and youthful. For chronic, widespread adult eczema, I encourage you to also explore what was touched on in the Beautiful Skin, Hair and Nails chapter, only if it resonates for you (I am referencing any rage that wells up toward a masculine figure in your life).

Fluid Accumulation at the Ankles

This indicates that the liver and/or the kidneys

need support. Do a four-week trial omitting caffeine; most people will notice a significant improvement in the fluid accumulation at the ankles in particular.

Newly Oily Skin and/or Oily Scalp

If greasy skin or a greasy scalp is new for you, it may signal that your sex hormones are imbalanced. This is particularly likely to be the case if you notice the greasiness increases in the lead up to menstruation. Utilize the sex hormone support strategies to see if that makes a difference.

Oily Skin at the Same Time as Dry Skin

Work on supporting sex hormone production; in particular, make sure that the pituitary gland is talking to the ovaries and that ovulation is occurring. Vitex can offer lovely support. Combination skin can also be a sign that the liver needs some love. Skin care may need to be changed to better support the skin's functioning.

Pale, Grey-Tinged, Dull Skin

This can be a sign of poor nutrition from poor food choices, or poor digestion. Focus on eating more real food if you don't already, and/or support your digestion through stress management and the other digestion strategies suggested.

Pigmentation on Face Newly Appearing

This can indicate a sex hormone imbalance.

Pimples and Blemishes

Based on where the blemishes tend to arise, use the insights in the Beautiful Skin, Hair and Nails chapter to decipher which body systems need support. For example, if blemishes always seem to appear along your jaw line, it can be a sign that your sex hormones need support. Do a dairy free trial for 4 weeks.

Psoriasis

Avoid pork and tomatoes for a trial period of four weeks. Essential fatty acid supplementation can be beneficial as can additional zinc. Enquire if you decided to "thicken your skin" to avoid emotional hurts.

Redness on the Face; Flush Easily

Commit to a dairy-free diet trail for four weeks.

Rosacea

Support the liver, and follow a strict dairy-free diet trial for a minimum of four weeks. You will notice significantly less redness by the end of this trial period if you are going to respond. Essential fatty acids can also be highly beneficial.

Scars

Consider taking additional vitamin C and/or zinc. Using lavender oil and/or calendula oil can also be beneficial to decreasing the appearance of scars.

Stretch Marks

They often indicate a zinc deficiency. You can also use lavender oil to minimize the appearance.

EATING HABITS

Inability to Stop Eating

Read *Accidentally Overweight*. Or, if this food behaviour started with a period of grief or other emotional turmoil, explore the following idea that is paraphrased from Geneen Roth, using grief as an example. If you are bowled over by grief, and your response is to eat a lot of cake, you halt your ability to move through the grief, as well as your confidence that it won't destroy you. If you don't allow a feeling to begin, you don't allow it to end.

Not Eating Enough

Explore with kindness and curiosity whose love, whose attention, you desperately want. And ask yourself: What would my heart have me do? Starve? No. What would courage have me do? Speak. Ask for help. Ask for a hug. It is never about the food or the lack of it. It is about how you perceive not eating enough makes you feel. But getting to feel the feeling you want to feel by depriving yourself of nourishment hurts your health and impacts on those around you. It is time to find other ways to feel the feelings that you want to feel, without hurting your health.

Often the root, as it is for so many situations, is a desire to feel loved. And once you find your path, you will naturally guide others to do the same. Now that's inspiring.

Struggling with Frustration

All emotions serve you. Emotions that you may think of as "negative" are merely calls to action. For example, if you feel frustrated, it may mean that you believe things could be better and they are not. This is a call to action, telling you there is something you could do now to make this better. This "negative" emotion is actually a gift if you use it effectively.

Struggle with Insecurity

As Steve Furtick so insightfully said: "If you struggle with insecurity, it may be because you are comparing your 'behind-the-scenes' with everyone else's highlight reel."

Relying on External Validation and Appreciation

When your shine relies on others telling you that you are beautiful, it can suggest that you no longer see or have an appreciation of your own beauty. When we hear a love song, we tend to think of others — either someone we love or someone who broke our heart. Try thinking about yourself during a love song. Direct the words into your own heart, letting them gently permeate the far reaches of your body, mind, and soul. Place your hands one on top of the other over your heart while you listen, if that appeals. Let yourself cry bucket-loads if that's what bubbles to the surface, for they will be tears of recognition for the precious beauty that you are. And you will see, or perhaps just catch a glimpse for a split second, that everything you have been searching for outside yourself — recognition, appreciation, compliments, people to love you — is within you. Always come home to that, to that beautiful love within you.

BEAUTIFUL WAYS TO SOOTHE BODY, MIND AND SOUL

Having shared numerous ways you can take great care of yourself, here are a few more just in case they appeal.

Beautiful Oils for a Bath

I am a huge fan of using certified organic or bio-dynamic skincare and bath oils. When I am asked to give examples of authentic beauty, I often say "women who radiate vitality and health". Their skin is clean and pure. Why? Plants are a big part of the answer. Most of their food, medicine, and skin care come from plants. What's more, the plants are pure, due to being grown in healthy soil, free from pesticides. Plants are a rich source of healing substances and vital energies. These life-giving plants are the basis for diet and skin care, and, hence, many aspects of beauty;and they are the basis of these beautiful certified organic and biodynamic oils, which are wonderful added to your bath. Many women love baths but rarely take them. Schedule time to do this at least once a week if you love them. If you are not a bath girl, then just using these plants as fragrances around the home can be uplifting or soothing, depending on what you feel like.

Lavender Oil

Lavender relaxes muscles and calms and soothes the nervous system. Any time you are under stress or on the edge of anger or fear, take a lavender bath to bring you back into balance and harmony or use the fragrance of the essential oil if a bath is not practical for you. Lavender cools hot skin conditions, such as inflamed capillaries and rashes. It relaxes and moistens dry skin, soothes nerves, and reduces redness and itching. Because it cools, lavender is great for hot summer nights. It is a perfect evening bath.

Lemon Oil

Essential oil of lemon refreshes and restores us when we suffer from physical exhaustion. Used as a healing tonic in virtually every culture, fresh squeezed lemon, or its essential oil, refreshes and tones the skin. Lemon juice or lemon oil is also used as an astringent to close oozing skin or treat rashes and allergies that cause too much moisture in the skin and sinuses. Lemon oil is an ideal bath for spring and summer.

Rosemary Oil

Rosemary promotes circulation. It warms, rejuvenates, and relaxes the body. Take a rosemary bath if you have chronically cold hands and feet (which can be a sign of oestrogen dominance and/or thyroid problems), or when you just can't get warm. I find rosemary is wonderful for people who do well with thyroid support. Rosemary also strengthens and warms the spirit. It is traditionally used if we feel weak, shy, or afraid, or suffer from metaphorically cold feet and simply can't face the world. Rosemary helps us relax when we have been working too hard for too long or feel overwhelmed by our problems. Rosemary is also used to treat sallow, listless skin because it brightens and restores colour. All of this makes rosemary ideal for an autumn and winter baths. Because it is energizing, if you like a morning bath it can be a wonderful way to start the day. If a bath is not practical for you, and you enjoy the fragrance of rosemary, you might like to keep a house plant. That way you can eat it easily, or you might like to just pull a piece from your plant, rub it between your fingers, and breathe in.

Sage Oil

Sage is used traditionally as a smudge (stick) to cleanse the spirit before sacred rituals. A sage bath can help neutralize hostile or negative thoughts and emotions, drawing out anger, fear, and sadness. It soothes and cleanses the internal rhythms of heavy or dark emotions and thoughts. A sage bath can also be used to treat body acne.

Spruce Oil

Spruce reins in emotions that seem out of control. It soothes and opens the lungs and the entire rhythmic system, restoring us when we feel emotionally exhausted, spent, or burnt-out. Spruce is an ideal bath for late winter and early spring, as well as whenever your lungs or sinuses are congested.

Calendula

I am a huge fan of the Calendula[4] plant. I love it used as a medicinal herb and also topically as an oil. I love it so much for the skin that it deserves a little section of its own. Here's why ...

Calendula officinalis is a highly regarded medicinal flower with bright yellow, gold, and orange blooms. Calendula is full of flavonoids, which are antioxidants found naturally in coloured plant foods such as vegetables and fruits; they give plants their lovely bright colours. Flavonoids protect the cells of the human body in much the same way as they do the plants, shielding them from free radicals and damage that can lead to disease and aging. Oil infusions made from calendula flowers have been traditionally used for the treatment of skin ailments and to facilitate wound healing.

---

4   Calendula oil is generally regarded as a very safe oil, but it is not suitable for people with allergies to the Asteraceae family of plants (such as daisies).

Calendula has anti-inflammatory properties, making it useful for stubborn wounds, skin inflammations, and varicose veins. It is effective in treating skin problems such as rashes, and, in particular, grazed and cracked skin, and is also useful for use when treating abrasions, sunburn, superficial and limited burns, insect bites, and even eczema.

Calendula oil is well known for its beneficial use on babies. This nourishing oil can be used for massage, moisturizing, or adding to bath water, leaving the baby's skin feeling soft and supple. It is suitable for daily care, and is an excellent product for cleansing and healing the nappy (diaper) area. Because of its mildness, calendula oil is beneficial for all people who have sensitive skin, not just babies. Calendula oil also makes a great base for lotions, creams, natural cosmetic products, and herbal ointments; it is also a common base oil used in aromatherapy.

Calendula oil can be used for treating venous complaints. In cases of venous inflammation, the ointment should be lightly applied, blending it with cypress and lemon essential oils. When applied consistently, this calendula oil combination has been shown to decrease the symptoms of varicose veins and venous congestion by inhibiting inflammation, toning tissue, and promoting enhanced blood supply to tissue.

Further benefits of calendula oil:
- ✓ It is an excellent remedy for soothing and moisturizing dry and chapped skin and lips.

✓ Due to its anti-inflammatory properties, calendula oil can be used for skin sores and inflammation, and to relieve the swelling and inflammation caused by bruises or muscle sprains. It can accelerate the healing of minor cuts, wounds, acne, burns, and insect bites.

✓ People with dermatitis, psoriasis, and eczema can also benefit from the topical application of calendula oil.

✓ You can use calendula oil for scars, or for preventing or reducing the formation of scar tissue.

✓ Calendula oil has been shown to increase collagen levels, which helps to prevent the formation of scar tissue.

✓ Calendula extracts have also been shown to help in treating haemorrhoids.

✓ Calendula oil helps soothe nipples that are sore from breastfeeding.

The Immense Beauty and Gift of Nature

The skin, like all of your organs, is infused with an energy that permeates all of its cells and gives it health and beauty. That underlying life force, as it is known in traditional medicine modalities, is intimately connected to your inner beauty. If you allow yourself, you can perceive this underlying life force when you touch your face, and experience your own light.

In traditional healing modalities, the connection between your hands and your spirit is very strong, so strong that it can make you forget the skin of your face or the bones beneath the skin when put your hands to your face. Do so with a feeling of wonder and gratitude. There is wisdom in wonder. By enhancing your connection to your inner life, your beauty can be experienced, firstly by you and then with anyone with whom you wish to share it.

Spending time in Nature strengthens that inner connection, as Nature's healing rhythms bring calm and renewal to our lives. Nature is not only an immense source of external beauty, but also a nurturing force that can restore physical and emotional health and beauty. Spend time in Nature observing, and feeling grateful, letting Nature's grace wash over you.

THE FINAL WRAP-UP

Beauty is a light in your soul. It is in everyone. It's just that, at some point, we stop believing in our own preciousness, our own beauty. But do you stop believing in the sun just because the moon has come out? Your beauty may momentarily disappear from your own view, but it is always there. It just gets clouded over by behavioural patterns, challenging life experiences, beliefs based on what others have said — which is a reflection of who they are, not who *you* are — and images and stories from the media. You just need to look and see what is getting in the way.

Your beauty is always present, yearning for you to believe in yourself again. You were born believing in yourself, your beauty, and the gold within you. You just forgot. But I want to encourage you with all of my heart to awaken that part of you that has gone to sleep. She may have gone to sleep with the part of you that takes such good care of you, including how you feed yourself, the thoughts you think, and how you tell yourself you have to be to be loved or liked or to fit in. Awaken that part of you that has gone to sleep, and love yourself the way the sun loves the earth. As Daniel Ladinsky so beautifully wrote:

Even

After

All this time

The Sun never says

To the Earth,

"You owe me."

Look

What happens

With a love like that.

It lights the

Whole

Sky.

Go light up the whole world with your radiance. xx

30 Essential Beauty Gems Online Course

My mission is to educate and inspire you and sometimes the spoken word does that powerfully.

I have created an online course called the *30 Essential Beauty Gems Video Programme*. During this course we explore your beauty pyramid and understand the five layers of beauty. The base layer explains the 12 Beauty Fundamentals, such as the layers of the skin, the ways we age and what it necessary for great hair… just to name a few! Then we have nine Beauty Challenges, which include fluid retention, pimples, skin congestion, acne, and backne. This is followed by the six Beauty Processes, including digestion and detox, as they are so critical to all beauty processes. As we approach the tip of the pyramid, I take you through the two Tell Tale Beauty Signs – what your eyes and face reveal - and we finish with one Beauty Belief.

I have created a 10 minute daily coaching video which you receive via email to ensure you stay focused on your inner health and desired beauty outcomes.

For more details visit: **www.drlibby.com** and the *Beauty from the Inside Out* resources page at:
www.drlibby.com/bioresources

Beautiful References
& Resources

Here I include additional information that may assist you on your journey. These are books and articles I have cited in the text, listed here if further reading in a particular area interests you.

Nutrition information is always changing, and I am passionate about keeping you up-to-date. I want you to have access to the latest and most insightful discoveries in health and well-being. Please be sure to visit my website and connect as a registered reader. This is a free service that allows you not to miss a thing! This service will also keep you informed about my live seminars, as I travel extensively and bring my message to life. It is my favourite thing to do ... other than write books!

After reading *Beauty from the Inside Out*, you may ask, what's next? I get many emails from people all over the world saying they feel like I have read their diary when it comes to describing how they feel in the pages of my books. People tell me that they want more of this type of information and a specific pro-gramme to follow that encompasses guidance around food and hormone balancing. They also want strate-gies that give them further insight into their emotional eating patterns. I cannot encourage you enough to check out the array of options on my website. Become a registered reader of *Beauty from the Inside Out* and get access to free beauty information and updates at: www.drlibby.com/bioresources

My mission is to educate and inspire people, and help them have an empowering relationship with their bodies, their health, and how they see themselves. I aim to put the power of choice back in people's hands.

So visit: www.drlibby.com to continue your *Beauty from the Inside Out* journey. I also post health information each day on Facebook, Twitter, and Instagram. Connect with me there at:

www.facebook.com/DrLibbyLive
www.twitter.com/DrLibbyLive
www.instagram.com/drlibby

It is an honour to assist you on your personal journey.

Not all of the areas presented in this book have additional resources listed, as I have read and studied widely (sometimes from very geeky biochemistry textbooks), and this book is the culmination of my knowledge, experience, observation, and intuition in this area to date.

Bays, Brandon. *The Journey.* London: Harper-Collins Publishers, 2004.

Bennett, Jane. *A Blessing Not a Curse: A Mother–Daughter Guide to the Transition from Child to Woman.* Bowral, Australia: Sally Milner Publishing, 2002.

Bennett, Jane, and Alexandra Pope. *The Pill: Are You Sure It's For You?* Sydney: Allen & Unwin, 2008.

Coates, Dr Karen, and Vincent Perry. *Embracing the Warrior: An Essential Guide for Women.* Burleigh Heads, Australia: Arteriol Press, 2007.

Deida, David. *The Way of the Superior Man.* Boulder, CO: Sounds True, 1997.

Epstein, Donny. *The 12 Stages of Healing.* San Rafael, CA: Amber-Allen Publishers, 1994.

Fasano, Dr Alessio *et al.* "Zonulin, a newly discovered modulator of intestinal permeability, and its expression in celiac disease." *The Lancet* 355: 9214 (2000) 1518–19.

Hay, Louise. *You Can Heal Your Life.* Carlsbad, CA: Hay House, 2004.

Horvath, K., and J. A. Perman. "Autistic disorder and gastrointestinal disease." *Current Opinions in Pediatrics* 14:5 (2002): 583–87.

Horvath, K, and J. A. Perman. "Autism and gastrointestinal symptoms." *Current Gastroenterology Reports* 4:3 (2002):251–58.

Horvath, K., *et al.* "Gastrointestinal abnormalities in children with autistic disorders." *Journal of Pediatrics* 135:5 (1999):559–63.

Jin, W. *et al.* "Increased intestinal inflammatory response and gut barrier dysfunction in Nrf2-deficient mice after traumatic brain injury." *Cytokine* 44:1 (2008): 135–40.

Mills, Simon, and Kerry Bone. *Principles and*

Practice of Phytotherapy. London: Churchill Livingstone, 2000.

Naish, Francesca. *Natural Fertility*. Bowral, Australia: Sally Milner Publishing, 1991.

Northrup, Dr Christiane. *Women's Bodies, Women's Wisdom*. London: Judy Piatkus Ltd, 1998.

Robbins, Anthony. *Awaken the Giant Within*. London: Simon & Schuster, 1992.

Roth, Geneen. *Lost and Found: Unexpected Revelations About Food and Money*. New York: Viking Penguin, 2011.

Weaver, Dr Libby. *Accidentally Overweight*. Auckland: Little Green Frog Publishing, 2011.

Weaver, Dr Libby. *Rushing Woman's Syndrome*. Auckland: Little Green Frog Publishing, 2012.

Weaver, Dr Libby and Tait, Cynthia. *Dr Libby's Real Food Chef*. Auckland: Little Green Frog Publishing, 2012.

West Kurz, Susan. *Awakening Beauty the Dr. Hauschka Way*. New York: Clarkson Potter Publishers, 2006.

Whitton, Tracy. *Stillness Through Movement*. Gold Coast, Australia: Tracy Whitton, 2011.

CDs

Weaver, Libby. *Restorative Calm*. Auckland: Little Green Frog Publishing, 2012.

Whitton, Tracy. *One With Life*. Gold Coast, Australia: Tracy Whitton, 2011.

Acknowledgements

Thank you, Chris Weaver, for all that you are. Thank you for being such a delicious human and husband and a superstar CEO. Thank you for being a visionary, and for your insights, your passion, your direction, your guidance, your courage, your authenticity, your humour, your arms, your love, and for delighting me. Thanks for being such fun and for your beautiful eyes and magical heart.

Thank you to my dear Mum and Dad, for your unconditional love and support, and for having parsley and chickens in the backyard. I am so blessed to have you for my parents and for the friendship that we share today.

Thank you to my delicious team: Kate, Imogen, Jenny, Dee, Annabel, and Leanne. Thank you for your contribution to the world through who you are and through your work. I miss you when I go away and always look so forward to seeing you. Sometimes it is hard to work; I love chatting and laughing with you so much! Super special thanks to Kate for her assistance with the research for this book, for her brilliant humour, her care, and her grace. Huge thanks to Imogen for her passion for beauty, her wonderful ideas, and her attention to detail. To Jenny, thank you for your wonderful knowledge of human biochemistry and herbal medicine, and also for your caring nature.

To Dee, thank you doesn't go close to conveying the enormity of my gratitude to you for overhauling our systems, for your calm and fun nature, and for the smile I can hear in your voice when you answer the phone. Thank you to Leanne, otherwise known as Amazeballs, thank you for your excitement, passion, insights, and deep care for my intentions in the world, and for helping me share these messages globally.

To the Real Food Chef team, chef Cynthia and Courtney, thank you for nourishing my body, mind, and soul with so many "situations of glory" while I created this book, and for cracking me up time and time again until my cheeks ached. #You'reJoking.

And thank you to the eWeb Marketing team whose passion for spreading happiness, success, and fun in the world is infectious and a joy to be part of.

Thank you to the beautiful humans who are my treasured friends, Karen, Leisel, Petrea, Alexandra, and Karloski, for the love, fun, music, film, insights, philosophies and beauty you bring to my life and to the lives of those you touch.

Heartfelt thanks to my beautiful-hearted editor, Caroline. Thank you for understanding my intentions in the world and for helping me craft this manuscript into what it is today. Thank you to Stasia, my super-clever designer, for the way she captures my sentiments with colour and images, and to Susan for her flexibility and layout skills. Thank you too, to Kate for her professionalism and invaluable touches to the final manuscript.

Thank you to the gifted and heart-centred humans, Jamila Cranston-Buckley, Steve Katz, and Tracy Whitton, who help care for my health. I am grateful for your care, your skills and our chats. And to Tash and Wai for being so great at what they do. I want to acknowledge Dr Rudolf Hauschka and Elisabeth Sigmund for their healing intentions for the world and for creating such magnificent skin care that nourishes both humans and the planet. Thank you for the most divine rose fragrance my senses have ever experienced.

Thank you to all of the farmers who grow our food and our skin-care ingredients, and who nurture the soil. I deeply appreciate what you do.

And to my three favourite little girls: Bella, Ruby, and Cedes. May you grow up always remembering, never doubting, that you are so delicious, so precious, and so very beautiful.

Meet Dr Libby

"My mission is to educate and inspire, enhancing people's health and happiness, igniting a ripple effect that transforms the world." — **Dr Libby**

Dr Libby Weaver, PhD, is one of Australasia's leading nutrition specialists and women's health experts. Dr Libby's passion for empowering people to make optimum health and lifestyle choices has led her to consult privately with individuals. She also consults in the corporate health arena, as well as with universities and the media. She has twice been a number-one bestselling author, and is a sought-after international keynote speaker. Her passion and insight inform and uplift audiences everywhere.

Dr Libby completed her PhD examining biochemical and nutritional factors in children with autism at the University of Newcastle, Australia. The outcomes of her PhD have affected the way the condition is treated in Australia and New Zealand.

It was through this work that Dr Libby came to better understand the role that various foods and hormones play in influencing our body shape and size, our appetites, our responses to exercise and stress, our clarity of thought, and our sleep patterns, and a host of other behaviours.

Working at Australia's leading health retreat where Dr Libby frequently shared these insights, Dr Libby's concepts were often described as "life-changing". She reaches a broad range of people, from businessmen and businesswomen and stay-at-home parents, to prominent sportspeople and Hollywood stars. Dr Libby's powerful messages are delivered through the pages of her bestselling books, *Accidentally Overweight, Rushing Woman's Syndrome*, and *Real Food Chef*, as well as through her informative live events and online training courses.

Dr Libby has become one of the most sought-after authorities on women's health. Through education and insight, Dr Libby encourages women to bring their bodies back into harmony naturally, and to understand the impact of emotions and beliefs on their biochemistry and behaviour. Her focus is on getting to the heart of nutritional issues and possible hormonal imbalances arising from modern-day life. She offers a refreshing and engaging perspective with real, sustainable solutions. Armed with abundant knowledge, scientific research, and a true desire to help others see their own light and beauty, Dr Libby empowers and inspires people to take charge of their health and happiness.

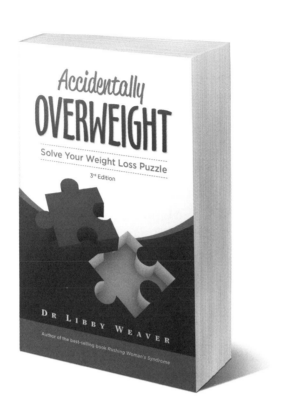

Accidentally Overweight

Accidentally Overweight, Dr Libby's first number-one bestselling book, identifies nine key factors within the body that directly impact on a human's ability to access body fat and burn it. These nine factors are: Calories, Stress Hormones, Sex Hormones, The Liver, Gut Bacteria, The Thyroid, Insulin, Alkalinity, and Emotions. Dr Libby clearly demonstrates how there is so much more to weight loss than the outdated calorie equation that sees weight as a simple reflection of calories in versus calories out.

So many readers say that *Accidentally Overweight* could easily be called "Optimal Well-being", as the information is relevant to everyone regardless of their health goals. Whether consciously or subconsciously, many people are frustrated by how they feel about their body, including sometimes its appearance, and this frustration can take up their headspace and influence their moods. Many people eat well and exercise regularly, yet their body fat does not reflect their efforts. Others have gained and lost the same 20 kilograms for the past 20 years. This book explains the biochemistry and emotions of weight loss to help free people from their battle with their bodies.

What to eat and how much to eat for optimum health and ideal body shape and size can seem like confusing and, at times, overwhelming areas to explore. Right now you could walk into a bookshop and pick up a book that tells you to eat plenty of carbohydrates, as they are essential for energy, and right beside it on the bookshelf will be a book that tells you not to eat carbs because they make you fat and tired.

How on Earth are you supposed to make sense of this well-meaning, but conflicting, information? How do you work out a way of eating that fuels you with great energy all day long while burning fat? What do you do if you feel like you have tried everything to lose weight only to gain it back? Have you ever put your mind to losing weight and made an enormous effort to eat well and exercise regularly for little or no reward? Or perhaps you are actually OK with your weight but you just don't *feel* right? *Accidentally Overweight* answers all of these questions, and more.

To learn more visit www.drlibby.com

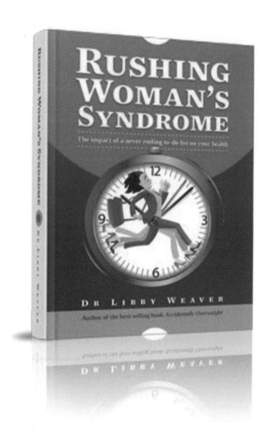

Rushing Woman's Syndrome

Hot on the heels of Dr Libby's first number-one bestselling book, *Accidentally Overweight*, Dr Libby's second book, *Rushing Woman's Syndrome*, became another number-one bestseller. *Rushing Woman's Syndrome* describes the biochemical and emotional effects of constantly being in a rush, and the health consequences that urgency elicits.

It doesn't seem to matter if a woman has two things to do in her day or 200; she is in a pressing rush to do it all. She is often wound up like a top, running herself ragged in a daily battle to keep up. There is always so much to do, and she rarely feels like she is in control and on top of things. In fact, her deep desire to control even the smaller details of life can leave her feeling out of control, even of her own self.

Rushing Woman's Syndrome examines the nervous system, endocrine system (including sex and stress hormones, the thyroid, and the pituitary gland), and the digestive system, as well as the emotional aspects of why women rush. Dr Libby can simplify even the most difficult biochemistry effortlessly, making this book equally educating and inspiring. What sets Dr Libby's work apart in a world where we are constantly bombarded with health messages, is her ability to search for, and explain, the underlying cause of an ailment, the why. *Rushing Woman's Syndrome* takes you on an emotional journey to help you decipher just where your beliefs are coming from and how those thoughts affect how your body behaves. So come on a journey of food and hormones, thoughts and perceptions, energy, and vitality. It is impossible not to see your life and body from a whole new perspective after reading this book.

Rushing Woman's Syndrome was inspired by Dr Libby's clinical experiences and her empathy for women and the many roles they now juggle. Dr Libby believes we have to be educated and inspired to make changes; her unique conversational style makes you feel like she is speaking right to you. Dr Libby combines two decades of personal experience, 14 years of university, and 15 years of clinical experience to offer you real solutions to both the biochemistry and the emotional patterns of the rush.

After a multitude of requests for coaching and requests from women who were too busy to read the book (!), Dr Libby created two 30-day video coaching programmes called The Rushing Woman's Syndrome Quick Start Course *and the* Condition the Calm Advanced Course, *which guide you on your journey from rushing back to calm. These courses have achieved phenomenal results with women across the world who are now enjoying life without the rush.*

To learn more visit www.drlibby.com

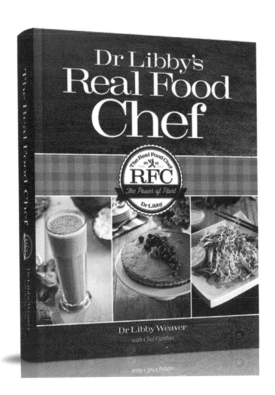

Real Food Chef

After noticing her clients struggling to come up with ideas for quick and nutritious meals, it seemed a natural progression for Dr Libby to create a series of recipes that have her seal of approval. And so the *Real Food Chef* was born.

The recipes appeal to a broad range of people, from busy mothers to teenage boys. Good, honest food that could be made by anyone; these recipes are sure to impress even the fussiest of eaters and offer nutrient dense alternatives to your favourite foods. From blueberry cheesecake to satay chicken, *Real Food Chef* is bursting with ideas and images to inspire.

The *Real Food Chef* system focuses on using food in its whole form, including all the food's vitamins and minerals and the natural plant compounds known to support human health; after all, it is nutrients that keep us alive. The recipes are free from refined sugars, dairy products, and gluten, with few exceptions; they are, therefore, suitable for those with some of the more common food allergies, or intolerances. Anyone who wants to optimize their nourishment would benefit from this book.

The *Real Food Chef* concept is a dynamic combination of Dr Libby's nutritional expertise with chef Cynthia Louise's gift for transforming everyday meals into nutrient-dense and incredibly delicious versions of their former selves. As a team, they bring you the why, and the how, to eat real food and amp up the nutrition in your world.

The *Real Food Chef* is a whole cooking system born from a desire to inspire you to eat low human-intervention food, real food the way it comes in Nature. Filled with delicious, nourishing recipes, quotes to inspire, and food education, the *Real Food Chef* is designed to enhance your quality of life and give you more energy to live the life you love.

We eat, on average, 35 times a week and these eating occasions supply the cells of your body with the nutrients to give you optimal health, energy, and vitality. So join this real food journey to discover how real food can revolutionise how you feel.

To help you create these incredible recipes, Dr Libby and chef Cynthia have returned to the *Real Food Chef* kitchen to show you how to make every dish in the *Real Food Chef Video Tutorials*. Chef Cynthia shows you step-by-step how to create your *Real Food Chef* masterpiece and Dr Libby provides the nutritional support, reminding you how each ingredient supports your body, mind, and soul.

To learn more, visit www.drlibby.com